Intraneural
Therapy
In Memoriam

12 April 1924 to 9 May 1988
Dr. Paul K. Pybus
M.A., M.B., B. Chir. (Cambridge), M.R.C.S., M.R.C.P. (London), D.R.C.O.G. (London),F.R.C.S. (England)

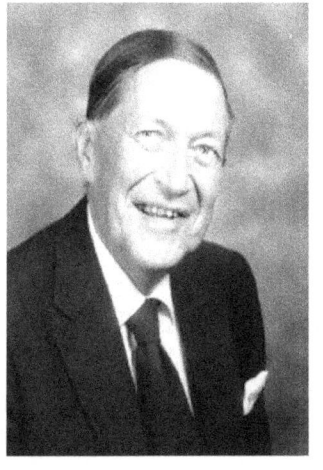

Paul was a wonderful man, filled with hope and energy and excited about this formation and successes of the Arthritis Trust of America (Rheumatoid Disease Foundation) officially titled "The Roger Wyburn-Mason and Jack M. Blount Foundation for the Eradication of Rheumatoid Disease, Inc."

The official title, you see, honored his mentor and friend Professor Roger Wyburn-Mason [M.D., Ph.D.], a man much respected by Dr. Pybus. Jack M. Blount, M.D. was one of the first two American physicians to consider seriously Wyburn-Mason's research, and to succeed in effectively treating Rheumatoid Diseases, Robert Bingham, M.D., was the other doctor.)

As founding member of the American "Rheumatoid Disease Foundation," Paul constantly sought with open mind to push us into challenging research opportunities. He contributed by his personal contacts with other physicians, medical studies, letters submitted to professional medical journals, letters to patients when requested, and in his generous attendance and clinical demonstrations at all of our medical conventions.

He was a founding member of The Rheumatoid Disease Foundation (American) and on the founding of this Foundation he went on to help establish the English and the Republic of South Africa counterparts.

Paul was a fighter, demanding honesty and integrity in the research and practice of medicine. He was that unusual physician who is willing to set aside prejudice and look anew.

As executive director and secretary of the Arthritis Trust of America, I found Paul more than just a very close friend and confidante but also a man who — as though he'd found a new and worthy goal — provided every kind of ethical support for this great hope for suffering arthritics.

Paul was a man who cared deeply!

He always gave full credit to Professor Roger Wyburn-Mason for his discoveries in intraneural therapies, but we all knew that Paul Pybus was the man who had taken a theory unimplemented and turned it into a golden bonanza for both Rheumatoid Arthritics and Osteoarthritics and other kinds of pains.

This publication, *Intraneural Therapy,* and the good results that have consistently stemmed from his work, are testimony to his brightness and desire to help patients in pain.

Kay Hitchen, formerly Executive Director/Secretary of the English Rheumatoid Disease Foundation, has this to say of her friend and teacher:

"Shortly after Charity status [similar to non-profit tax-exempt status] was granted to the South African branch, we were stunned to hear of the death of The Rheumatoid Disease Foundation's Chief Medical Advisor, Dr. Paul Pybus.

"Dr. Pybus studied at Cambridge and was houseman to Professor Roger Wyburn-Mason nearly 40 years ago; which was the begining of a life-long friendship that was to continue even after Dr. Pybus emigrated to South Africa in the 1950's.

"He was in regular contact with the Professor, and continued his work into the use of [Wyburn-Mason's] medicines to treat Rheumatoid Arthritis.

"Dr. Pybus developed his own technique of intraneural injections to bring relief from arthritic pain. A technique which he shared freely with any physician who wished to know of it. This method is now in use widely throughout the U.S.A. and also at our New Hope Clinic in Southampton, England. [New Hope Clinic no longer functions: Ed.]

"Although we had been [corresponding] for some years, I did not actually meet Dr. Pybus until The Rheumatoid Disease Foundation's first board meeting in the U.S.A. in 1983 and was overwhelmed by his kindness and professionalism, his desire to 'fly the flag' and maintain the British 'stiff upper lip'

Original publication for physicians
Intraneural Injections for
Rheumatoid Arthritis and Osteoarthritis & The
Control of Pain in
Arthritis in the Knee
by
Dr. Paul K. Pybus
M.A., M.B., B. Chir. (Cambridge), M.R.C.S. M.R.C.P. (London),
D.R.C.O.G. (London), F.R.C.S. (England)

From the Editor:

This foundation has long advocated the use of both prolo therapy (also called proliferative, sclerotherapy, or reconstructive therapy) as well as intraneural injections. Our founding health professionals, including Dr. Pybus, initially believed that the two therapies -- Intraneural Injections and Prolo therapy -- could not be administered simultaneously as prolo therapy acted by creating inflammation in specific positions while intraneural therapy acted to dampen inflammation in specific positions.

Those physicians who have routinely used both therapies have found this assumption to be untrue — which makes sense considering that the key words in each therapy are "specific positions."

We now hold that so long as the injections are not in or near to each other that both prolo and intraneurals can be used simultaneously.

We also invite the reader's attention to our website at http://www.arthritistrust.org.

Anthony di Fabio

Note:

The formula in this book originated by Dr. Pybus is stronger than it need be according to many doctors presently using Intraneural Injections. Some doctors now recommend the following:

To 50 ml vial of 1% lidocaine add 1 ml of a depot steroid such as Aristospan or Celestone Soluspan.

Some, including Drs. Curt Maxwell and Gus J. Prosch, Jr., M.D., have learned that Pybus' recommended depot steroid is totally unnecessary to achieve the same good results.

Apparently there's wide latitude for the practitioner in that several different mixtures have worked successfully.

"He always encouraged us when we were setting up the Foundation in England; that was at a time when the Professor [Wyburn-Mason] had just died, his wife [Joan] was grieving and it seemed as if David [Hitchen] and I were the only people in the country who wanted the Foundation to exist. Dr. Pybus was always writing, or sometimes phoning, from South Africa to remind me, 'of course we can do it — Good God, We're British!'

"He was a true British gentleman, who was also a gentle man which is why his patients loved him dearly.

"I will never forget his humour, and sense of 'fair play'.

"David and I have lost a great friend; his loss to The Rheumatoid Disease Foundation is immeasurable."

A brief resume' of Dr. Paul K. Pybus' experience and education follows:

Internship, St. Mary's Hospital, Paddington; House Surgeon to Obstetric Unit, Mr. Alex Bourne; Service in the Royal Air Force, 1948; Discharged with rank of Squadron leader 1950; House Physician to Professor Roger Wyburn-Mason, 1951-52; House Surgeon at Royal Cancer Hospital, London. Also worked with Roger Wyburn-Mason, 1951-52; Senior Medical officer, Battersea General Hospital, London. Surgical and Orthopaedic Registrar, St. Alban's Hospi- tal Hertfordshire, 1953-54; Surgical Registrar, Torbay Group of Hospitals, England, 1954-57; Proceeded overseas to Dares Salaam, Tanganyika and then to Nakuru War Memorial Hospital, Nakuru, Kenya, 1957. Emigrated to South Africa. Senior Surgeon, Edendale Hospital, Pietermaritzburg, Natal. 1962; Principal Surgeon, South West Africa Group of Hospitals, Windoek, 1973. Commenced general practice and rheumatology in Pietermaritzburg, Republic of South Africa, 1977. Chief Medical Advisor, Rheumatoid Disease Foundation, 1983 through May 9, 1988.

Dr. Paul K. Pybus serendipitously but independently discovered the effect of intraneural injections on certain key neuromata in the treatment of Osteoarthritis and Rheumatoid Disease, as based on theories taught by Roger Wyburn-Mason thirty years earlier.

The Arthritis Trust of America feels that this booklet, *Intraneural Injections* is a must for all forms of arthritits and arthritis-like pain, and that the use of designated intraneural injections decreases the time to wellness, regardless of what other modalities are used on the patient.

Englishman Roger Wyburn-Mason, M.D., Ph.D., nerve specialist, was the first to describe the causation principle of joint damage from tender nerve locations, sometimes called "trigger points," in arthritis and arthritis-like pain.

South African Dr. Paul K. Pybus, his former house physician, learned to implement in clinical practice Wyburn-Mason's theories of intraneural injections, successfully using his discoveries for more than 20 years.

American Keith McElroy, M.D. independently discovered the same principles, and applied them to his patients, also for many years.

Dr. Paul K. Pybus and Gus J. Prosch, Jr., M.D. explored additional key "trigger points," until it became clear to them that a virtual one-to-one correspondence existed between painful neuroma and acupuncture points -- but not always so.

Dr. I.H.J. Bourne, a friend of both Dr. Roger Wyburn-Mason and Dr. Paul Pybus, also developed the use of intraneural injections which he published as "Musculoskeletal Disorders: Local Injection Therapy."

Specialists in musculoskeletal pain have long used area-wide; i.e., non-specific "trigger points," intraneural injections and intra-articular injections, as well as nerve blocks to relieve pain. In other words, although their medical territory was not really inclusive, they unwittingly discovered some of the same points for patient pain relief. At the suggestion of Dr. Curt Maxwell, we recommend the W.B. Saunders book, *Atlas of Pain Management Injection Techniques* by Steven D. Waldman, M.D., J.D. as an excellent supplementary book. (It is very convenient for doctors who are into reimbursement via insurance, as it gives the insurance code that is acceptable for each of the injections.) The artwork is excellent, and there can be no doubt as to how to inject in the various parts of the body. The text is quite appropriate, giving not only the how, but also contra-indications, et. al.

Of most importance, however, for more than 50 years American Harry H. Philbert, M.D. independently developed the use of intraneural injections which he called "Specific Injection Therapy," covering many of the same aspects as the publications reported above. *The Anatomy of Pain: Specific Injection Therapy*, is a well-done report of Dr. Philbert's research.

Dr. Philbert's work will shock most medical practitioners, as he claims through his techniques alone to have improved the lot of many painful patients, and, in particular, has easily cured bronchial asthma, and other conditions, including some coronary problems. We're very sorry to report that we don't know where to purchase this extremely fine book.

Thanks are due Tony Chapdelaine, M.D. , M.PH.and Gus J. Prosch, Jr. M.D. for their review of the materials included.

Perry A. Chapdelaine, Sr., Ex. Dir./Sec
The Arthritis Trust of America

Introduction

This is a book written not only at the request of many physicians who would like to relieve pain in their many arthritic sufferers, but also at the special request of the Arthritis Trust of America/The Rheumatoid Disease Foundation, who have adopted this method of treatment for both rheumatoid and osteoarthritis.

Its use in osteoarthritis is quite dramatic and extremely useful and may even he curative for the nerve lesions, which I believe to be the cause of the condition. In the case of rheumatoid arthritis, however, it is also useful, but mainly as a 'first aid' procedure; it cannot he regarded as curative, as the real cure is with the anti-microorganism drugs and other causative factors.

The idea was originally formulated by my old friend and tutor, Professor Roger Wyburn-Mason, and it was he who first gave me the idea of treating arthritis joints in this manner. He would many times turn round and say, 'You know, I have a nice way of treating this', and would then show me these amazing techniques that would normally startle anyone with the minimum of medical knowledge. I asked him what our colleagues thought of this, but to this question he would only answer that they did not understand and had so many other interests. This I found difficult to believe at the time, but I have since realised the difficulties he must have had; as an example, I record his efforts to get recognition of his very simple method of treating most cases of 'sciatica. a condition that most people were then treating by laminectomy and removal of the intervertebral disc of 'L4, 5 & S1, with very mixed successes. His unpublished article forms Chapter IV of this book.

During my career as a general surgeon with occasional turns of general practice, I would encounter the odd case of failed laminectomy for prolapsed disc and then I would treat with alcohol injections with good results. It was not, however, until I entered full-time general practice that I got the opportunity of treating many arthritic cases, and, remembering Wyburn-Mason's teaching, I was able to develop his ideas further, so that I am now in the position of being able to relieve any joint pain that is presented to me. This is a possession of undoubted value to any doctor and it is described here for the use of anyone who would like to possess this gift. It is a gift that is unsurpassed in its value and the joy it gives, not only to patient, but also to the doctor as he sees the surprised look on the joyfully, amazed patient who has suffered pain and frustration for so long. It is a means of doing real good to mankind.

These techniques are readily demonstrable, and I should like to thank The Arthritis Trust of America/Rheumatoid Disease Foundation, not only for publishing this book through the enthusiasm of Perry A. Chapdelaine, the Executive Director to the Foundation, but also for the opportunities they have given me to demonstrate the techniques on others. You too can do this and likewise startle your colleagues. Good luck to you all!

Dr. Paul K. Pybus, M.A., M.B., B. Chir. (Cambridge), M.R.C.S., M.R.C.P. (London), D.R.C.O.G. (London),F.R.C.S. (England)

INTRANEURAL THERAPY

by

Paul K. Pybus, MB, FRCS (Eng.)

[Late Principal Surgeon, South West Africa Group of Hospitals Late Senior Surgeon, Edendale Hospital, Pietermaritzburg General Practitioner and Rheu- matologist, Pietermaritzburg.]

CHAPTER 1

The idea of interfering with peripheral nerves has always been to all doctors an austere concept. We are always taught in our student days, and with good reason, to leave nerves severely alone, as interfering with these delicate structures can cause a great deal of distress, pain and paralysis. This is indeed true for many procedures such as surgery, injections of sclerosing agents or severe heat as produced by coagulating diathermy.

But there may now be no fear of permanent side effects, as in our form of intraneural therapy only a very dilute solution of Triamcinolone Hexacetonide (Lederspan or Aristospan) is instilled into the nerve, the diluent being 1/2% of a local anaesthetic. Thus, if a motor nerve should be involved, and this is most unusual, then any motor paralytic effect quickly wears off and the patient can go home after a short waiting period.

Thus it is very reasonable for any practitioner of average competence, a reasonable proficiency with a syringe and a fair knowledge of anatomy, particularly of the superficial nerves, to perform all the procedures described in the following few chapters.

It is a technique well worth learning and becoming proficient in. Not only is it comparatively painless but the results are most gratifying both to the patient and to the medical attendant.

TROPHIC NERVES

For many years toward the end of the last century and in the beginning of this, the existence of trophic nerves was largely accepted as serving a protective role for the tissues. They were, however, of minute dimensions, and this eventually led to their very existence being challenged and, as a result, largely ignored.

Futhermore, the occurrence of indolent ulcers seen in denervated areas of the skin was in those days fairly common. Unfortunately, they were called 'trophic ulcers', a badly chosen name as they were now subconsciously attributed to trophic nerves, the existence of which was coming to be doubted. In the absence of any substantial scientific proof of their existence, they became lost in the morass of rapid advancement of medical scientific proof that occurred at that time. That these ulcers should really have been named 'atrophic ulcers' will be apparent from what follows.

CONDUCTION OF PAIN

There are two types of pain experienced by the human body, namely:

1. **Epicritic or superficial pain**. This is a pain such as is produced by a pinprick and is conducted by the Aδ-type fibres, or type III of the American classification. These fibres are thick, having a fibre diameter of 5µ m and a rapid conduction rate of 30 metres per second, and are myelinated to produce a slow anaesthetisation rate of 5 minutes. They arise from receptors in the skin, are relatively few in number and have their cell bodies in the dorsal horn of the spinal cord. These fibres are rapidly fatigable and play no part in the production of arthritic pain.

2. **Protopathic or deep pain.** In contrast to the above, this is the deep pain experienced in inflamed tissues such as joints, and is conducted by the C-type fibres, or type IV of the American classification. These fibres are thin, having a diameter of 0.5µ m and a slow conduction rate of 1 metre per second, and are unmyelinated to produce a rapid anaesthetisation rate of 2 seconds. They arise from pain receptors in all the deep and superficial tissues, are very much more numerous than the A fibres and have their cell bodies in the ganglia of the dorsal roots. These fibres are responsible for the production of arthritic pain and are identical with the trophic nerves as described by Wyburn-Mason.

These C-fibres are responsible for reflex responses and are, unlike the Aδ fibres, only slowly fatigable. In this discussion we will refer to them by their older name of trophic nerves.

These trophic nerves originate from both superficial and deep organs of the body and are ubiquitous. When irritated anywhere along their length they can transmit ectopic impulses in both forward (prodromic) and reverse (antidromic) directions. Prodromic impulses produce the sensation of slow pain by conduction of impulses along the branch axons of the posterior root ganglia cells into the cord and thence to the brain. In addition, as they are also responsible for reflex actions, they relay in the ventral horn cells to produce an out-flow into the muscular fibres, resulting in a reflex muscular spasm. The anti-dromic impulses pass to the blood vessels and other structures in the region of the peripheral origin of these nerve fibres, causing the liberation of the peptide SP (Substance P, a Neurohormone), leading to the increase of the blood[2,3,4] supply, heat and oedema in these situations being the changes of inflammation. Liberation of SP also occurs when the distal end of a freshly cut sensory nerve is stimulated in both man and animals.

Sir Thomas Lewis' showed that a mild noxious stimulus to intact skin resulted in the 'triple response'. This consists of a local area of capillary vasodilation surrounded by one where the fluid contents of the blood have leaked out through the permeable capillary walls, and this again surrounded by an area of local arteriolar vasodilation or 'flare'. These are the fundamental changes of inflammation in miniature. The ease with which this response is induced varies with the subject's emotional state and the presence or not of neurological or mental disease (Tache ce're'brale), itself indicating the importance of centrifugal (antidromic or reverse) nervous impulses in the modification of the 'triple response'. Lewis showed that experimental section of the posterior nerve root supply to the affected area and its subsequent degeneration modified the 'triple response' by abolishing the flare, and the same abolition will be assumed to occur in the full-blown inflammatory response to a stimulus by suppression of 'antidromic' posterior nerve root impulses.

It has long been recognised that the condition of causalgia is due to some partial damage or section to a sensory nerve. In this condition a mild stimulus, which produces little or no reaction on normal skin other than the triple response, will induce a grossly excessive inflammatory response in the painful parts affected by the causalgia,[6,7,8,9] and what is more, this response persists in this region and even proceeds to cellulitis. Warm water may cause excessive inflammation whilst mustard plaster blisters it more readily than in normal areas. This is due to the excessive nervous activity from trophic nerves and results in extreme inflammation.

In contrast, complete section of the nerve to any area of skin renders it anaesthetic and any damage to this area results not in inflammation but in necrosis and the formation of a so-called 'trophic ulcer', really an atrophic ulcer. There is no attempt at healing or regeneration. This is seen in anaesthetic areas from syringomyelia in the hands, tabes dorsalis in the feet, in paraplegics or in the anaesthetic areas of skin caused by leprosy. The same is true of anaesthetic areas produced by sciatic nerve section in the dog. Furthermore, if mustard oil is placed near such a sore it results not in inflammation, pain or even a triple response but in a further area of painless gangrene with no attempt at healing.

The lens of the eye is the only living organ in the body that has no nerve supply and is never subject to inflammation after injury but rather to necrosis.

Malignant tumors have no nerve supply. It has been shown by Wyburn-Mason[10] that trauma or the application of substances which normally produce inflammation, such as nitrogen mustard, to malignant tissues produce not inflammation but necrosis in them, and hence the use of these drugs in treatment of malignancies.

Local anaesthetic rapidly depresses activity in these trophic nerves; if it is applied to them, the nervous activity is abolished and so is any inflammation in the tissues supplied by these nerves.

Not only local but general anaesthetisation can also depress this nervous activity, as was shown in one of Wyburn-Mason's personal cases. He quoted a case of identical twins, both suffering from rheumatoid arthritis, both taking the same anti-inflammatory drugs and both deteriorating to the same extent. Then suddenly one brother started to improve and the reason for this was not realised until it became apparent that he had found that he got relief from the pain by sniffing cocaine snow, and he was now an addict! His twin brother, however, continued to deteriorate. The cocaine was obviously acting as a suppressant of trophic nervous impulses and so causing symptomatic resolution of the disease.

It must be seen that trophic nerves do exist, or to put it another way, the C-type unmyelinated nerve fibres have a trophic activity, and suppression of this activity leads to resolution of inflammation, whilst complete abolition of the same impulses produces necrosis when the anaesthetic tissue is damaged.

ELECTRICAL POTENTIAL IN NERVES

It is a well-known fact, described in most textbooks of physiology, that in a normal resting nerve there is a definite electrical potential difference of approximately -70 millivolts between the inside semi-fluid contents, which have a negative charge, and the outside of the nerve, which is positively charged. This is shown in Figure I.

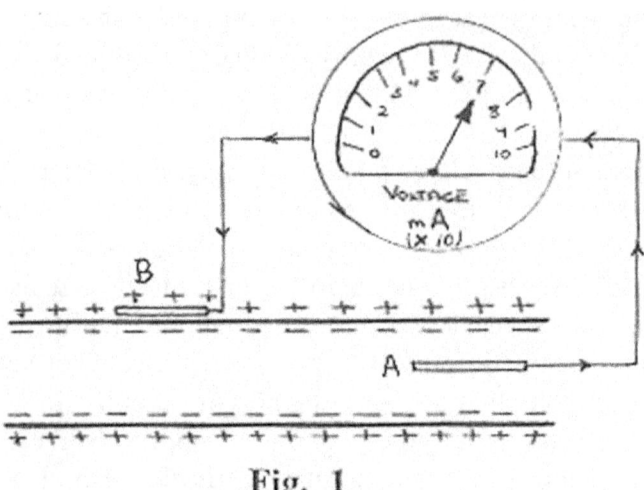

Fig. 1

At the terminal end of a trophic nerve (C-type unmyelinated fibre) is a plain nerve ending or terminal button, and these terminal buttons are sensitive to external stimuli initiating a destabilisation of the neurilemma in which the nerve fibre is enclosed.

This destabilisation results in the escape of electrons or negatively charged particles through the nerve membrane to neutralise the positive-charged outer surface. This causes further destabilisation along the nerve, resulting in an on-going leak of electrons, so that the impulse is propagated in this fashion.

Normally impulses are only conducted along the nerve in this prograde fashion, as the membrane is rapidly restabilised after the passage of the impulse and is restored to its resting state, when it is again ready to receive another impulse. The time between the passage of the impulse and restoration to normality is in the region of 2 milliseconds and is known as the latent period. This period is divided into an absolute refractory period, during which time no stimulus, however strong, will produce an impulse, and a relative refractory period during which a stronger-than-normal stimulus will produce an impulse. In this way, if the impulses are strong enough it is possible to produce a barrage of impulses which summate one with another to produce a tetanus.

Normally impulses are only initiated at the endings of an axon, but if this axon is stimulated anywhere along its length the stimulus creates a small area of destabilised membrane and an area of negativity due to a leakage of electrons through the membrane to the outer surface. On this area of negativity impulses are propagated in both directions, namely, prodromic and antidromic. Figure 2. The prodromic impulse is relayed to the dorsal horn of the spinal cord and is conducted to the brain, where it is interpreted as pain. In addition, it is also relayed through the spinal reflex to the local

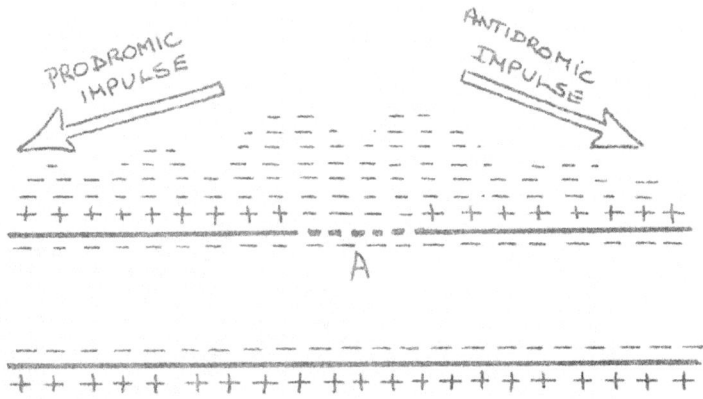

Fig. 2

musculature to produce a contraction, and the part is removed from the supposed painful stimulus.

The antidromic impulse is conducted peripherally where it produces SP substance to cause vasodilation of the capillaries, and this in turn produces a leakage of fluid from the dilated capillary into the interstitial tissue.

16

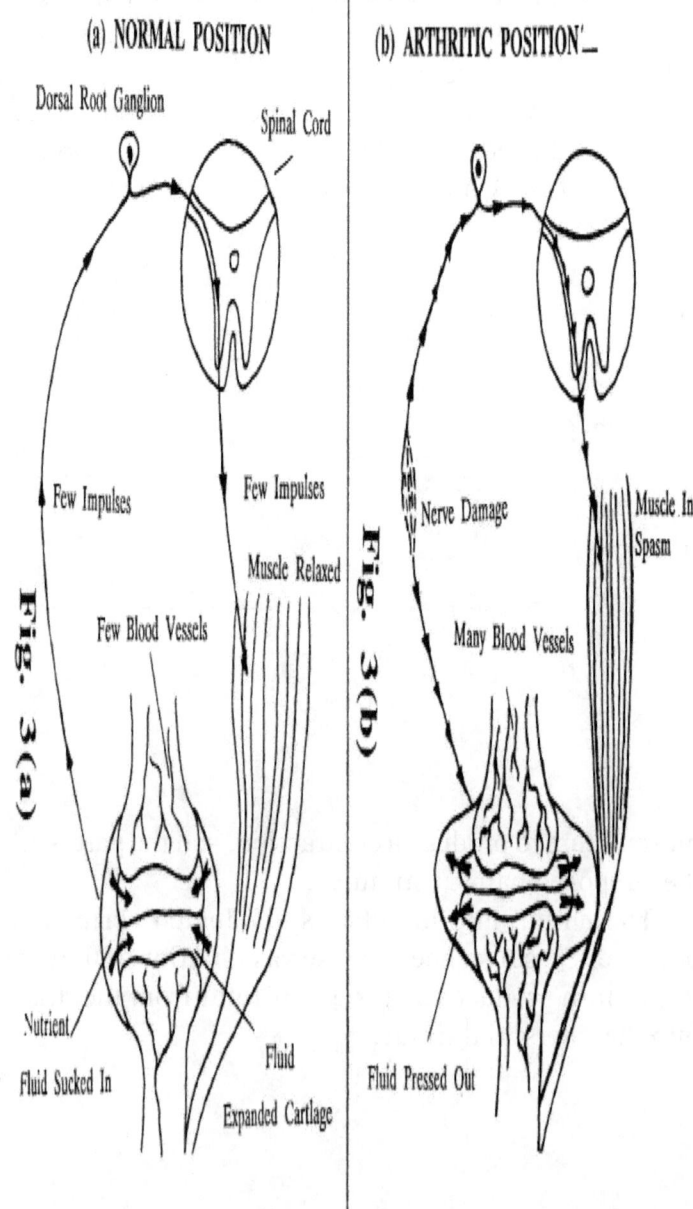

(a) NORMAL POSITION (b) ARTHRITIC POSITION—

Dorsal Root Ganglion

Spinal Cord

Few Impulses

Few Impulses

Muscle Relaxed

Few Blood Vessels

Fig. 3(a)

Nutrient

Fluid Sucked In

Fluid

Expanded Cartlage

Nerve Damage

Muscle In Spasm

Many Blood Vessels

Fig. 3(b)

Fluid Pressed Out

EFFECT OF DAMAGE TO THE TROPHIC NERVE

Let us take the argument a stage further. Suppose that instead of receiving a mild stimulus the axon is damaged in a place along its course between the cell and its receptor button. Then this produces a greater leakage of electrons through the traumatised sheath, causing a series of impulses to be set up; these summate to give a barrage of impulses. As the damage is in the course of the nerve fibre, these summated impulses are conducted in both an antidromic and a prodromic direction as described previously.

The antidromic impulses will be conducted peripherally to the region of the sensory nerve ending, where summated impulses to the blood vessels will cause intense dilation, local increase in temperature, oedema and even synovial effusion or, in other words, the changes of inflammation or osteoarthritis.

The prodromic impulses will be conducted centrally to the spinal cord where they relay in two main directions, namely:

1. To the spinothalamic tract to reach the thalamus where they are interpreted as pain. This causes the most annoying symptom but does not affect the joint in any way.

2. To the dorsal root ganglia and via intermediary neurons to the ventral horn cells which discharge to give a tetanic barrage of impulses to the local musculature.This will result in continous stimulation of all muscles in the area, producing a muscular spasm or stiffness and resultant compression of the joint surfaces as shown in Figure 3.

Thus, if the argument is so far understood, we have five conditions pertaining, namely:

1.a destabilised nervous membrane due to trauma with an electrical disturbance,

2. a distal inflammation due to antidromic inpulses,

3. referred pain in this joint from prodromic impulses arising in the damaged nerve and not in the joint,

4. reflex spasm of the musculature

5. compression of the articular cartilage.

We will now consider the last of these:

18

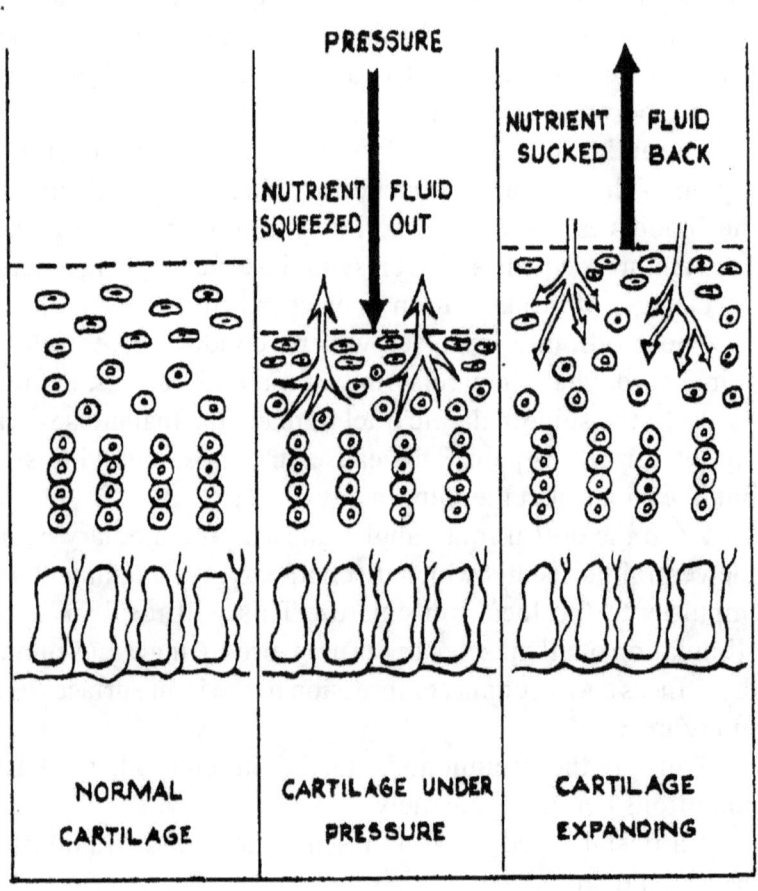

Fig. 4

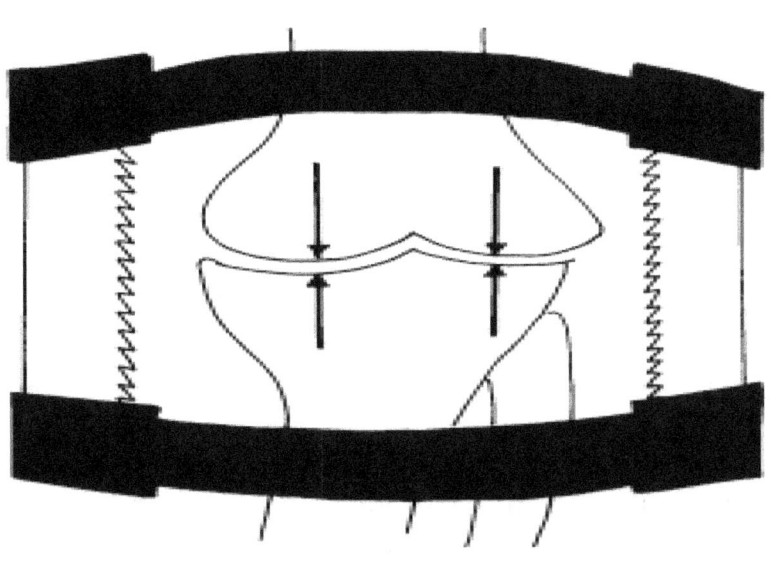

Figure 5. Charnley's clamp applied to the knee of a monkey to produce an osteoarthritis lesion.
The direction of force is shown by the arrows.

NUTRITION OF JOINT CARTILAGE

There are no blood vessels in healthy cartilage. The hyaline cartilage of joint surface consists of large cells arranged in palisades and suspended in a semi-fluid, resilient matrix which is compressable and expandable. The synovial fluid circulates in this semi-solid matrix and its circulation is maintained by alternate compression and reactive expansion of the cartilage. Thus as pressure is increased, as in weight bearing, the fluid is expressed out of the cartilage and the waste products of cellular activity are removed, and as the weight is taken off the joint surface the cartilage absorbs the fluid, bringing oxygen and nutriment to the cartilage. The cartilage acts like a sponge; this was described by McCutchen in his classical description in 1962, and is shown diagramatically in Figure 4. The only other source of nutrition for these cells is direct diffusion from the blood vessels of the vascularised bone marrow at the base of the cartilage which is inadequate.

Thus nutriments and oxygen are received and waste products removed mainly by the process of alternate expression and soakage of fluid as described, apart from the small amount that diffuses directly from the blood vessels at the base of the cartilage.

EXPERIMENTAL PRODUCTION OF OSTEOARTHRITIS

Osteoarthritis, or degenerative joint disease, has been produced experimentally in the knees of rhesus monkeys and rabbits by a number of workers over the past two decades. Salter and Field,[12] Trias[13], Crelin and Southwick[14] all performed experiments that were similar in their approach in applying continuous joint fixation and compression of the cartilaginous surface of the knees of these animals by means of the use of a Charnley clamp. Figure 5. An osteoarthritic-type lesion, including prominent cartilage degeneration, was produced in the joint following as few as three days of continuous fixation compression, and by the end of 14 days the condition was well established. After six weeks the joint degeneration was in its final stages, the cartilaginous joint surface being worn away with eburnation of the underlying bony layers. It was also shown by Callandruccio and Gilmer[15], that if experimental fixation and compression is released, the condition is reversible and the cartilage shows signs of regeneration. These workers

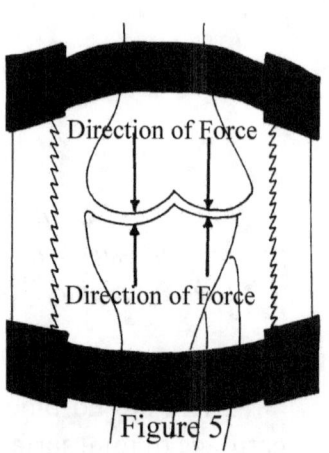

Figure 5

postulated that constant fixation compression of the joint surfaces acts by impairing the nutrition of the cartilage cells. This can be readily understood when it is realised that the circulation of the synovial fluid can no longer take place. The cartilage now solely depends on the nutrition brought in from diffusion from the vascularised bone marrow at the cartilage's base, and, this being insufficient, the result is death and disillusionment of the most superficial cells. Thus it can be seen that compression is a powerful factor in the production of osteoarthrosis by virtue of its curtailment of the oxygen supply to the cartilage.

If we accept this explanation it will be seen that the treatment for osteoarthritis or osteoarthrosis now becomes obvious. The root cause of the trouble is, therefore, not in the joint as previously presumed, but in the damaged destabilised nerve, and for relief of this condition treatment must be directed at this nerve.

As described previously, this area is negatively charged due to the constant leak of electrons, and for the nerve impulses to be stopped these excessive electrons have to be eliminated. This can be done in three main ways:

1. **Physical.** Use of acupuncture needles. These needles are made of resilient metal with a good conductivity of electricity. They are pointed, and when inserted into the body near an area of electrical charge will act as a miniature lightning conductor, the electrons being attracted to the point of the needle, and then distributed to the exterior via the hands of the operator, and thence to the earth, Figure 6. For three thousand years this principle of acupuncture has been practised in China, and for some time now western medicine has sought an explanation for its undoubted efficacy. The author, for one, has witnessed the efficiency of this method on numerous occasions when performed by others, and has also obtained similar results himself. He has also observed that the results are superior when the needles are deliberately earthed, as can be done by the simple method of removing the shoe of the operator.

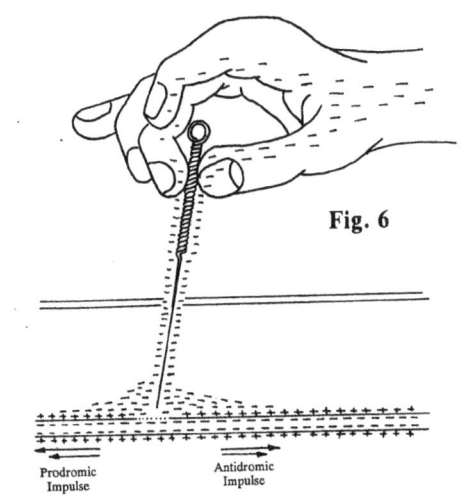

Fig. 6

Prodromic Impulse

Antidromic Impulse

Acupuncture, however, shows no great permanency in the relief afforded just by one treatment, as when the needle is removed the membrane is still destabilised and the condition reverts to the status quo ante.

2. **Chemical.** Local anaesthetic. Local anaesthetic is a well-known nerve stabiliser and its action is described in numerous textbooks of anaesthesia[16] -- all nervous impulses are blocked and none can be propagated. In the case of the C-type fibres or trophic nerves, this blockage of impulses takes a matter of two

seconds due to the lack of a myelin sheath (with the A fibres it takes a matter of minutes for the local to penetrate the thick myelin sheath).These two facts are well-known to anyone who has both performed regional anaesthesia by means of nerve block and injected so-called 'trigger points'' with a local anaesthetic agent. However, it is also well-known that neither the regional anaesthesia nor the relief of pain by local anaesthetics only is permanent; they last just as long as the anaesthetic stays in relation to the nerve or 'trigger point'. A further substance is required in order to stabilise the nerve more permanently.

3. **Healing agents. Corticosteroids or other anti-inflammatory agents**.The breach in the nerve sheath has to be stabilised permanently by the healing process and the inflammation eliminated. The most efficient of the anti-inflammatory agents is still cortisone. This has not been satisfactory in the past due to the undesirable effects when given by mouth. However, if this substance could be delivered at the site of inflammation in such a manner as to be permanently static in that position, then the desired effect would be achieved. Depo-steroid preparations are the present best solution to this problem. There are at least three of these available at the present time.

a. Triamcinolone hexacetonide (Lederspan or Aristospan). This has the advantage of slow absorbability and rapid action in producing diminution of inflammation in three to four hours. It is the ideal preparation at the present time.

b Betamethasone acetate (Celestone-Soluspan). This is also effective in two to three hours, but, unfortunately, the commercial preparation has the disodium phosphate salt also included, and as the latter moiety is rapidly absorbed there are dangers of resultant side-effects.

c.Methylprednisolone acetate (Depo-Medrol or Depomedrone). This also has a Depo effect but has the disadvantage that it takes six to eight hours for its anti-inflammatory action to take place. Thus there is a two to three-hour time lag between the action of the local and that of the steroid and therefore a period when the pain seems to recur with the fading of the local anaesthetic action; this period may be unduly prolonged.   It is possible that if a non-steroidal anti-inflammatory drug could

be made in a depot form suitable for injection intraneurally, then the steroids could be eliminated completely in treatment.

Unfortunately, to date no such preparation has been developed. (1984)

The peripheral nerves themselves in all parts of the body are supplied by small unmyelinated nerve fibres which pierce the perineurium with the blood vessels and are distributed to the nerve fibres within (nervinervorum)[9].

When these minute nerves are stimulated by trauma it will produce an inflammatory reaction in the nerve, which in turn stimulates the fibres in the main nerve, and it is then obvious that suppression of inflammation in this area will reduce all trophic activity in that nerve, with the consequent abolition of excess nervous impulses, thus breaking the vicious circle.

This can be done by the use of steroids, which are the most powerful anti-inflammatories on the market today. And it would explain their early success in the treatment of rheumatoid arthritis, even if the mechanism was not at the time fully understood. Later, due to the complications of this therapy, and to the large doses that were administered to get any result, it fell into serious disrepute, where it has rightly remained, even if it is still given, with definite indications, by some rheumatologists.

The collapse of the cortisone charisma, which was to cure all cases of rheumatoid arthritis, was followed by the development of non-steroidal anti-inflammatory drugs which acted by suppressing all inflammation throughout the body but had no steroid effect. These drugs, after an initial success, were also found not to be without their complications, causing a great deal of gastric upset with ulceration, gastric haemorrhage which was sometimes fatal, leucopoenia and even cases of agranulocytosis which were often fatal. They were, however, more acceptable than cortisone, as they did not cause the serious hormonal and electrolyte disturbances produced by the latter, and so now are largely the standard treatment (1984) [now methotrexate, even more dangerous].

However, both of these treatments have the same radical disadvantage, namely, their generalised action, when in point of fact the drug action is only required at the damaged site in the nerve.

During the dispute that was going on over the use of corticosteroids and of non-steroidal anti-inflammatory drugs, a number of very excellent products were produced for injecting into the joints with the idea of introducing the steroid where required, namely, the joint surface, and with the general absorption being kept to the bare minimum. These have had a variable success rate. Hollander[17], in the United States claims excellent results, but this treatment is by no means universally successful in other hands. Furthermore, it does not treat the root causes of trouble but merely the symptoms, namely, the inflammation of the joint; it ignores the primary nerve involvement.

The author has developed the idea of introducing an anti-inflammatory drug at the damaged nerve site. This anti-inflammatory would have to be slowly absorbed, and the only such injectable depot forms available at present are steroidal in nature. These are:

1. Triamcinolone hexacetonide (Aristospan or Lederspan)

2. Methylprednisolone acetate (Depo-Medrol or Depomedrone)

3. Betamethasone acetate (Celestone-Soluspan)

At present, as previously noted, no non-steroidal anti-inflammatory drugs are made in depot form, but such a drug, if available, would be extremely useful.

It will be seen that the local anaesthetic stabilises the nerve in the first five hours, and meanwhile the depot steroid is healing the traumatised breach in the nerve membrane. Thus, when the local has worn off the membrane is largely healed and normality is restored.

All the various joints have definite points where nerves tend to be damaged around them. These points, if inflamed, have the properties of a neuroma, namely:

1. They are tender to the touch,

2. They are all in the anatomical line of a known nerve,

3. They are painful on distortion,

4. They are rapidly eliminated by a number of physical means, viz:

    a. Insertion and grounding of an acupuncture needle[18],

    b. Local application of various physical agents such as cold, heat, massage, short wave, ultrasound, etc.,

    c. Injection of local anaesthetic and depot steroid as described.

The technique of injection and the position of these points will be described in the next chapter.

REFERENCES

1. Wyburn-Mason R, **Trophic Nerves**. Henry Kimpton. London 1950:305

2. lgnelzi RJ, Atkinson J H, *Pain and its modulation: I, Afferent mechanisms*. Neurosurgery 1980;6:577-583

3. Wright S, **Applied Physiology**, 9th edition. Oxford University Press 1952:721

4. Iversen DI, Iversen LL, *Substance P. A new central nervous system transmitter*. Hospital Update 1981;5:497-506

5. Lewis T, **Blood Vessels of the Human Skin**. Shaw and Co. London 1927

6. Charcot JM, **Lecons sur les Maladies du Syste'me Nervaux.** Delahaye et cie. Paris 1875;1

7. Mitchell SW, Moorhouse CR, Keen WW, **Gunshot Wounds and Other Injuries of Nerves**. Lippincott and Co. Philadelphia 1864

8. Gowers WR, Taylor J, **Diseases of the Nervous System**. Third edition. Churchill and Co. London 1899

9. Wyburn-Mason R, Trophic Nerves. Henry Kimpton. London 1950

10. Wyburn-Mason R, **The Reticulo Endothelial System in Growth and Tumor Formation.** Henry Kimpton. London 1958

11. McCutchen CE, *Animal joints and weeping lubrication*. New Sci- entist 1962;15:928-930

12. Salter RS, Field P, *The Effects of continuous compression of living articular cartilage: an experimental investigation*. Bone and Joint Surgery 1960;42A;31-45

13. Trias A, *Effect of persistent pressure on the articular cartilage.- an experimental study*. Bone and Joint Surgery 1961;43B:376-386

14. Crelin EX, Southwick WD, *Changes induced by sustained pressure in the knee joint articular cartilage of adult rabbits*. Anat Rac 1964;149:113-134

15. Callandruccio RA, Scott GW, *Proliferation, regeneration and repair of articular cartilage of immature animals*. Surg 1962;44A:431-455

16. Wylie WD, **A Practice of Anaesthesia.** Lloyd Duke (Medical Books) Ltd. London; 41:1157-1159 Dripps RD, Eckenhoff JE, Vandam LD. **Introduction to Anaesthesia**. WB Saunders and Co. London 1972;16:213-216

17.   Hollander JL, Brown EM, Jessar RA, *Hydrocortisone and cortisone injected into arthritic joints: comparative effects and use of hydrocortisone as a local antiarthritic.* J Amer Med Ass 1951;147:1629-1635

18. Pybus PK, *Nerve membrane stabilisation.* Brit Med Acupuncture Soc J 1984;16

CHAPTER II

THE MANAGEMENT OF INDIVIDUAL PAINFUL JOINTS

As explained in the previous chapter, rheumatoid disease is not primarily present in the joints but in certain local peripheral nerves, and the arthritis is only a secondary but painful manifestation of the condition. Each arthritic joint involved has situated round it several local areas of destabilised nerves, and these points are to be described later as to their location. Initially the management of the typical joint will be considered.

TECHNIQUE OF INTRANEURAL INJECTIONS

The treatment of all arthritic joints is exactly the same. The joint is first assessed clinically as to shape, colour, swelling, temperature, degree of pain and function. It will also be observed that the joint is still and the muscles in spasm, and on attempting movement creaking or crepitus is elicited. The joint is next palpated with a definite intent in view by means of a prodder (the eraser end of a pencil or even the thumb of the operator is usually adequate for the purpose) along the course of known nerves, and certain positions of intense tenderness will be noted. Proceed as follows:

1. Mark the most tender spots with a skin pencil.

2. Raise an intradermal bleb of 2% local anaesthetic. The author uses Mepivacaine but any form of local anaesthetic is suitable. This can be done with a needle and syringe, but a Dermojet injector is quicker for the operator and less painful for the patient, and is generally more acceptable. The Dermajet was introduced to the missionary field by Robert Hingston, working in Nicaragua. It earned the name of 'Pistola de la paz', or, 'the gun of peace', due to its success in the rapid vaccination technique developed in that country, and later to be accepted world-wide, resulting in the eventual elimination of smallpox. [Mada-jet : Mada Medical Products, Inc., 625 Washington Ave., Carlstadt, N.J. 07072, in U.S.A.; or use an internet search to find other companies.]

3. Make up a mixture of 1/2% local anaesthetic and 0.5ml of a deposteroid in a 10ml syringe.

4. Introduce the needle of the syringe through the anaesthetic bleb and aim in the direction of the suspected position of the nerve, meanwhile keeping a close scrutiny of the patient's facial expression.

5. When the needle reaches the position of the damaged nerve a sharp pain is experienced, and at this precise time the patient's facial expression will change and the operator will know at once that he is in the correct place. This is far more accurate than awaiting the patient's complaint of pain or even a verbal outburst, which may occur when the needle has pierced through the other side of the nerve and so the injection could be given too deep.

6. The mixture is now injected into this exact tender spot. This is most important and is the secret of the technique. It is a method of accurately delivering the steroid in the position where it is most wanted; it will remain there semi-permanently.

7. Once the needle is withdrawn no further pain is experienced, and each other marked spot is similarly treated until all the neuritic areas are no longer tender.

8. Each injection site is now covered with a small dry dressing as they tend to bleed, probably due to the local release of prostaglandins.

9. The joint is now put through all possible movements, and it will be immediately obvious, not only to the patient but also to the doctor, that there is now no longer any pain and the joint is much looser; in fact, it will be felt to loosen up 'just as if oil had been injected into the joint'. More mechanically-minded patients will often volunteer this observation. The crepitus is also noted to be less marked.

10. The patient now uses the joint and is surprised to learn that there is no longer pain and his range of movement has been greatly increased.

Each joint, or group of joints, will now be described in detail with special references being made to the individual nerves involved.

A. THE SHOULDER

The main nerves involved in the shoulder joint are:

a. Circumflex (axillary) nerve
b. Suprascapular nerve
c. Supraclavicular nerve

a (i). Axillary nerve

This is a branch of the posterior cord of the brachial plexus (C5 and 6). In passing back it pierces the deep fascia, where it can be traumatised by this fascia, giving the first injection point. The needle

28

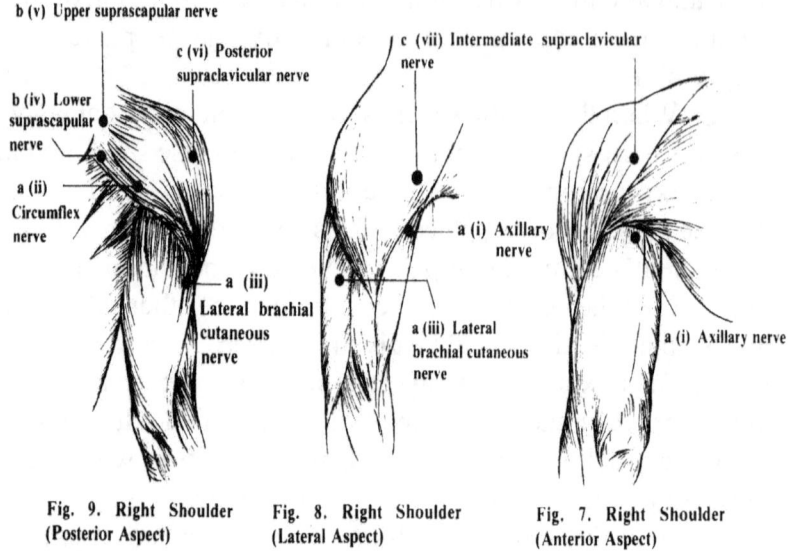

Fig. 9. Right Shoulder
(Posterior Aspect)

Fig. 8. Right Shoulder
(Lateral Aspect)

Fig. 7. Right Shoulder
(Anterior Aspect)

is introduced at the lower end of the anterior axillary fold and directed laterally until pain is experienced and the injection is made. (Acupuncture nomenclature: Heart 1). Figures 7a (i).

a (ii). Circumflex nerve

This nerve passes back in close relation to the lower part of the capsule of the shoulder joint, piercing the fascia in the quadrilateral space. It gives a branch to the capsule of the shoulder. The needle is introduced between the teres major below and the teres minor above, and the triceps laterally. The needle is directed forward until pain is experienced and the injection made. [Acupuncture nomenclature: Small Intestine 9). Figures 9a (ii)]

a (iii). Lateral brachial cutaneous nerve

This is the continuation of the circumflex nerve when it pierces the deep fascia in the postero-lateral part of the upper arm. It is pinched in the fascia and is often noted to be tender. The needle is introduced over the tender spot and advanced medially and slightly forwards till the tender spot is reached and the injection made. [Acupuncture nomenclature: Large Intestine 14). Figs 8a & 9a (iii)]

b (iv). Lower suprascapular nerve

This is a branch of the upper trunk of the brachial plexus which enters the supraspinous fossa and passes around the base of the scapular spine, where it can be abraided by the scapular movement.

Introduce the needle below and medial to the acromion, and pass the needle forward and slightly laterally and upwards till the bone of the base of the spine is felt and pain is experienced as the nerve is entered. Inject about 1 ml of mixture. [Acupuncture nomenclature: Small intestine 10). Figures 9h (iv)]

b (v). Upper suprascapular nerve

Occasionally this nerve has to be approached from above the scapular spine, from the supraspinatus fossa, and is again encountered at the base of the scapular spine. [Acupuncture nomenclature: Small intestine 12). Figures 9b (v)]

c (vi). Posterior supraclavicular nerve

This is a branch of the cervical plexus and is injured over the lateral point of the shoulder when an injection is often made to inject the subacromial bursa. I consider that this nerve is often silenced by this procedure. [Acupuncture nomenclature: Large intestine 15). Figures 9c (vi)]

c (vii). Intermediate supraclavicular nerve

This is also a branch of the cervical plexus and often tender on the joint line, but anterior and below the posterior branch, and the nerve is just deep to the skin. [Acupuncture nomenclature: Lung 1). Figs 7c (vii)]

In any case of arthritic or painful shoulder all the above points are sought and ONLY IF TENDER are they marked on the skin with a skin pencil, and treated as described.

At the conclusion of treatment the shoulder is put through its full range of movements and usually these are free and painless. If, however, the movements are still painful it may be necessary to treat a few other spots in the region, but these cases are the exception rather than the rule.

B. THE ELBOW

There are four nerves involved in the elbow joint which are:

a. Lateral antebrachial cutaneous nerve

b. Medial antebrachial cutaneous nerve

c. Posterior antebrachial cutaneous nerve

d. The nerve to anconeus muscle.

a.Lateral cutaneous nerve to the forearm

This is the termination of the musculocutaneous nerve, a branch of the lateral cord of the brachial plexus, C5,6,7, which, having pierced the coraco-brachialis, runs down laterally between the biceps and the brachialis muscles to reach the lateral side of the

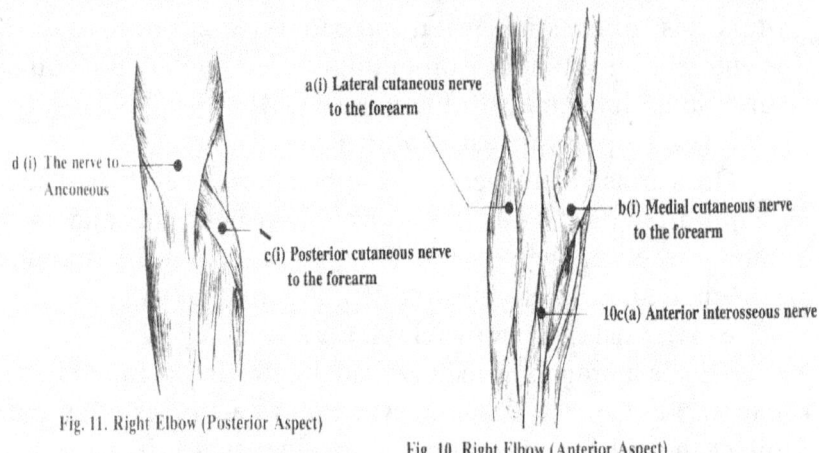

Fig. 11. Right Elbow (Posterior Aspect)

Fig. 10. Right Elbow (Anterior Aspect)

arm, and, below the elbow, pierces the deep fascia over the brachioradialis, to become the lateral antebrachial cutaneous nerve. It is at this point where tenderness is found, and treatment of the tender area produces instant relief of pain in the elbow. Figure 10a(i) (Acupuncture nomenclature: Lung 5). When injecting this nerve it is possible that the needle can be introduced too deeply and the radial or posterior interosseous be also injected to produce a temporary wrist drop. This is only a transient embarrassment to the doctor and patient as it quickly passes off. The patient should be accompanied by a driver if he is in charge of a motor vehicle!

b. Medial cutaneous nerve to the forearm

This is a branch of the medial cord of the brachial plexus, C8, T1 , and runs on the medial side of the brachial artery, piercing the deep fascia with the basilic vein in the arm. At the elbow-joint level it divides into two branches and here it is often tender; injection can be done at this point medial and superficial to the brachial artery. However, this point like all others is only injected if tender, and is not so universally tender as the lateral cutaneous nerve to the forearm. Figure 10b(i) [Acupuncture nomenclature: Heart 3].

c. Posterior cutaneous nerve to the forearm

This rises in common with the lower lateral cutaneous nerve to the forearm, perforates the lateral head of the triceps and descends along the lateral side of the arm posterior to the lateral epicondyle, where it may be involved. If tender this is also injected. Figure 11C (i) [Acupuncture nomenclature: Large Intestine 12].

d. The nerve to Anconeous

This nerve is also a branch of the radial in the spiral groove and passes down to the anconeous. It is occasionally tender superior and lateral to the olecranon. Figure 11d. (i) [Acupuncture nomenclature: Triple warmer 11.]

These four points are described for completeness, but the main one is the lateral antebrachial cutaneous nerve, the others being secondary and only comparatively rarely involved in advanced cases. Many cases of 'tennis elbow' are often confused with this form of neuritis and are relieved by the injection of the nerve.

C.THE WRIST

This joint is usually controlled when treatment is given for the hand and fingers (see later); however, should the patient still have pain in the wrist apart from the hand and fingers, then the wrist can often be contolled by injecting the anterior interosseous nerve which gives the nerve supply to thisjoint. This point can be found in the line of the nerve as it is given off from the median nerve below the level of the pronator teres. Figure l0c(a). (Acu- puncture nomenclature: Pericardium 4).

D. THE HAND AND FINGERS

Control of the arthritic hand is one of the most dramatic beneficial effects of intraneural therapy. The nerves involved are:

a. Posterior interosseous nerve (for the fingers and hand)

b. Terminal branches of the radial nerve (for the thumb)

c. Dorsal branch of the ulnar nerves (for the little fingers.)

a. Posterior interosseous nerve

This is a terminal branch of the radial nerve, C5, 6, 7, 8 and T1 roots, and after piercing the supinator, which it supplies, it then descends on the posterior surface of the interosseous membrane to reach the back of the carpus, where it presents as a flattened enlargement or 'ganglion' from which fine neural filaments are distributed to the ligaments and the articulation of the carpus.

These filaments would appear also to be distributed to all muscles and tendons of the hand and fingers, as in every case of the painful arthritic hand this ganglion, lying as it does between the tendons of extensor digitorum and extensor digiti minimi, is exquisitely tender. Furthermore, if it is infiltrated with local anaesthetic and depo-steroid the result is immediate and semi-permanent relief of all pains and spasm in all of the muscles and joints of the hand and fingers. puncture nomenclature: Triple warmer 4).Figure 12(a) [Acupuncture nomenclature: Triple warmer 4]

b (i). Medial terminal branch of radial nerve to thumb

This is situated just lateral to the tendon of extensor pollicis longus. Figure 12b(i) [Acupuncture nomenclature: Large Intestine 5].

b (ii). Lateral terminal branch of radial nerve to thumb

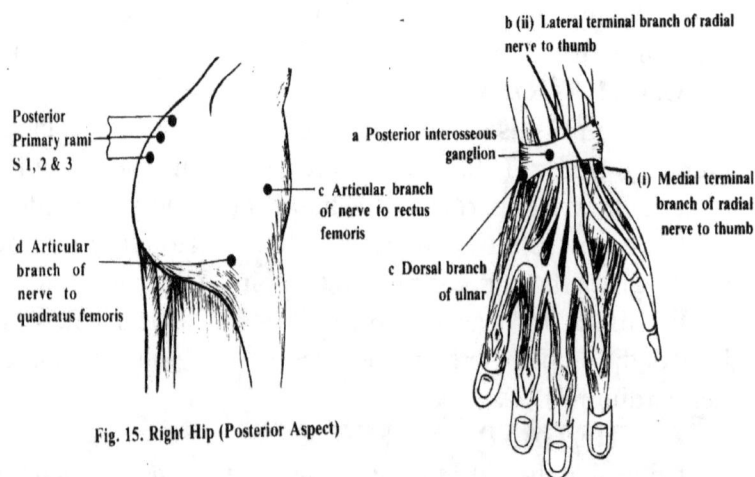

Fig. 15. Right Hip (Posterior Aspect)

Fig. 12. Right Hand & Wrist (Posterior Aspect)

This is slightly lateral to the above and is shown in Figure 12b(ii). [Acupuncture nomenclature: Lung 9].

c. Dorsal branch of ulnar nerve (for the little finger).

Occasionally these first two points do not completely relieve all pain, especially the little finger. The Dorsal branch of the Ulnar can be found to be tender on the medial side of the wrist, just posterior to the pisiform bone. Injection at this point will often relieve pain in the little finger. [Acupuncture nomenclature: Small Intestine 5. Note joints on diagram. Figure 12.

E. The Hip

Regional hip blockade has been described elsewhere by an anaesthesiologist who developed the technique for the relief of intractable pain due to osteo-arthritis of the hip that for some reaso or another, was unsuitable for surgery. [4,5,6,7] The nerves involved are as follows:

a. Obturator nerve

b. Lateral femoral cutaneous nerve

c. Nerve to rectus femoris

d. Nerve to quadratus femoris

a. Obturator nerve

This nerve is usually regarded mainly as a motor nerve supplying principally the adductor muscles of the thigh. It does, however, give off both cutaneous and articular branches which are often traumatically inflammed.

a (i). At Obturator's entrance to the thigh through the obturator foramen

Blocking at this point is described by James and Littleffi,[4]. This point of tenderness is below the pubic tubercle and medial to the femoral vein. A long needle is used and directed medial to the femoral vein, passing backwards to hit the bone and then worked inferiorly until pain is experienced and the injection made. Figure 13a (i). [Acupuncture nomenclature: nil].

a (ii) Articular branch of the posterior branch of the obturator nerve

This runs laterally to the medial side of the greater tuberosity and is tender at this spot. The author injects this point with a long needle introduced in front and medial to the point; it has to be introduced deeply and when pain is experienced the injection is made. 5 ml is usually required. Figure 14a(ii). [Acupuncture nomenclature; nil].

b. Lateral femoral cutaneous nerve

L2, 3 and 4 passes through the origin of the sartorius muscle to enter the thigh and it is here that its branches, of which there are usually two, are damaged causing spasm of the muscle and fixed flexion. Blocking of the nerves often abolishes so-called fixed flexion of the hip, which is probably in reality spasm of the sartorius muscle. Figure 13b [Acupuncture nomenclature: Gall bladder 27].

c. Articular branch of nerve to rectus femoris

This rises from the posterior division of the femoral nerve and gives a twig to the hip joints which runs laterally under cover of the upper part of the greater tuberosity. It is once again better approached obliquely from above the tuberosity. Figures 14 & 15c. [Acupuncture nomenclature: nil].

d. Articular branch of nerve to quadratus femoris

This is a branch of the sacral plexus. The articular branch of the nerve to rectus femoris passes laterally from the parent trunk and is also better approached obliquely from behind with a long needle. Figure 14 and 15d. [Acupuncture nomenclature: nil].

After these injections the hip is put through full movement, and Thomas' test for fixed flexion is repeated and the result compared with that prior to treatment. Also, increased abduction is often most evident due to injection of the obturator nerve in the groin. Figures 13a(i).

F. THE KNEE

Injury to the knee occurs when the knee is slightly flexed and is one of forced abduction and external rotation; this will result in a tearing of the medial longitudinal ligament, and of necessity the overlying saphenous nerve in the angle between the tibial condyle and the shaft of the tibia. Figure 16. This point is the main area of damage in the lower limb and is tender in nearly all cases of lower limb sprain or damage. The chief nerves involved are:

a. The saphenous nerve and its branches
b. The external femoral cutaneous nerve
c. The intermediate femoral cutaneous nerve
d. The external femoral cutaneous nerve
e. The peroneal nerve
f. The medial femoral cutaneous nerve
g. The posterior femoral cutaneous nerve.

a (i). The saphenous nerve

This is found at the angle described above. Palpate the medial border of the tibia and pass the finger upwards towards the tibial condyle to where a tender spot is found. Raise a bleb at this point and direct the needle upwards and slightly laterally, until the point is found and the injection made. Two (2) ml is usually required here. Figure 16 & 17a(i). [Acupuncture nomenclature: Spleen 9].

a (ii). Origin of the infrapatellar nerve

As the surface markings of the nerve are followed upwards and

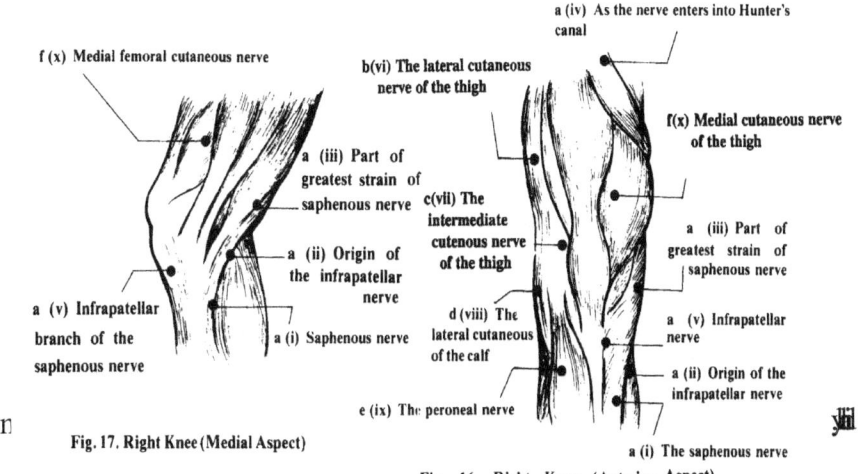

Fig. 17. Right Knee (Medial Aspect)

Fig. 16. Right Knee (Anterior Aspect)

a further tender spot is located medial and above the previous site. The needle is directed upwards and laterally, and the injection made. Figures 16 & 17a(ii). [Acupuncture nomenclature: Liver 7].

a (iii). Part of greatest strain of saphenous nerve

The surface markings of the nerve are again followed upwards and backwards from the previous point and tenderness is elicited just on the joint line. From here the needle is directed laterally until the tender spot is found. Figures 16 & 17a(iii). [Acupuncture nomenclature: Liver 8].

a (iv) As the nerve enters into Hunter's canal

This point is quite deep and the needle is directed backwards. Fig. 16a(iv) [Acupuncture nomenclature: Spleen 11]. This point is often found in women, but very rarely found in men due to the increased angle of the female pelvis.

a (v). Infrapatellar branch of the saphenous nerve

This is also tender and can he located over the upper medial surface of the tibia just below the knee.Figure 16 & 17a(v). [Acupuncture nomenclature: nil].

b(vi) The lateral cutaneous nerve of the thigh

This is damaged and is tender as it pierces the fascia lata 5 cm above the knee on its lateral aspect. The needle is passed medially and the point found. Figure 16 & 18b (vi) [Acupuncture nomenclature: Gall bladder 32]

c(vii).The intermediate cutaneous nerve of the thigh

This is often found to be tender at the upper and lateral corner of the patella. The point is easily found and injected. This is often the site chosen for aspiration of the knee, which may explain the extreme pain experienced when the manoeuvre is inexpertly performed. Figure 16 & 18c(vii). [Acupuncture nomenclature: Stomach 34].

d (viii). The lateral cutaneous nerve of the calf

This nerve may be tender but usually only in the more severe and advanced cases. It is a branch of the lateral popliteal nerve and perforates the deep fascia over the lateral ligament of the knee. It is simply approached as it is subcutaneous. Figure 16 & 18d(viii). [Acupuncture nomenclature: Bladder 53].

e (ix). The peroneal nerve

This lies between the two peronei muscles and is here often tender. It is a favourite spot for the acupuncturist. Figure 16 & 18e(ix). [Acupuncture nomenclature: Stomach 36].

f(x). Medial cutaneous nerve of the thigh

This nerve is also occasionally involved and is tender medial and superior to the patella. The injection is made fairly deeply at the tender spot. Figure 16 & 17f(x). [Acupuncture nomenclature: Spleen 10].

g(xi). Posterior cutaneous nerve of the thigh

This nerve is the only point that is worth injecting on the back of the knee. It is situated where the nerve perforates the deep fascia of the thigh and is sometimes tender. The injection is made very superficially at the tender spot. The needle must not be introduced deeply for fear of damage to the popliteal vessels. Figure 19g(xi).

As can be seen, there are many nerve points around the knee, and these have been found at different stages over an eight-year experience in this field. Far the most constant point is that of the saphenous nerve at the angle of the shaft and medial condyle of the tibia, known as Spleen 9 to the acupucturist; it has been described regularly in the medical literature over this period[8,9].

It has since been mfound that for constant good results the others also exist and require treatment. It is again stressed that only tender spots are to be treated: for effectiveness of the injection, the nerve must be both inflammed and, therefore, tender.

G. THE ANKLE AND THE FOOT

Once more it can be observed that sprains to the ankle and foot are again those of external rotation and abduction. If the force is very great it will result in an external rotation fracture of the ankle, and the same strain that damages the knee. This would explain why the brunt of the damage affects not only the ankle and foot, but also the knee, as described elsewhere[10].

The main nerve involved, therefore, is the saphenous nerve. The nerves are enumerated as follows:

a (i). Saphenous nerve

This is invariably tender a little below the main knee point on the tibial shaft. Here the needle is directed almost laterally and the tender nerve injected. Figure 20a (i). [Acupuncture nomenclature: Spleen 8].

a(ii). The examining finger is now moved down along the anterior border of the tibia, and three-quarters of the way down a tender spot is often found. Reference to anatomy books will show the presence of a constant branch at this point.[11] This requires only a minimum of injection fluid. Figure 20a(ii). [Acupuncture nomen- clature: Liver 5].

a(iii). The finger is run down a little more and a further spot is found just below, where a second constant branch comes off the saphenous nerve. Fig- ure 20a(iii). [Acupuncture nomenclature: Spleen 6].

a (iv). The saphenous nerve is also found tender anterior to the medial malleous in close relation to the great saphenous vein. Figure 20a(iv) [Acupuncture nomenclature: Liver 4]

b. Superficial peroneal nerve, medial branch

This nerve is also found to be tender over the dorsum of the ankle joint. The point is fairly deep and lies on the dorasal ligament of the ankle. Figure 20b. [Acupuncture nomenclature: Stomach 41].

c. Sural nerve

The sural nerve is also often tender and is associated with pain under the foot. It is found between the Achilles and peronei tendons. Figure 21c. [Acupuncture nomenclature: Bladder 60.

Summary

In this chapter I have tried to enumerate and describe the various tender nerve points. They are all places where the nerve tends to be traumatised; and, in summary, the following points are stressed:

1. Only tender places should be injected.

2. The Depo-steroid is diluted to the extent of 1/20 in 0.5% local anaesthetic. This gives maximum coverage of the nerve with fine particles of insoluble steroid.

3. Between 1-5ml of this liquid is injected according to the site and the area to be covered.

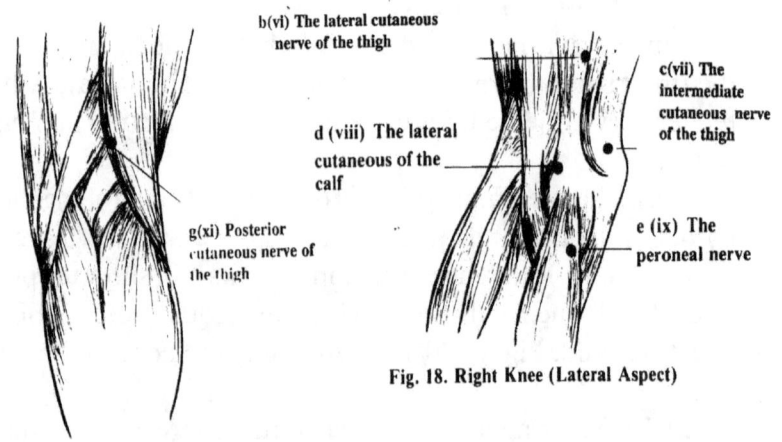

b(vi) The lateral cutaneous nerve of the thigh

d (viii) The lateral cutaneous of the calf

c(vii) The intermediate cutaneous nerve of the thigh

g(xi) Posterior cutaneous nerve of the thigh

e (ix) The peroneal nerve

Fig. 18. Right Knee (Lateral Aspect)

Fig. 19. Right Knee (Posterior Aspect)

4. There is almost invariably more than one spot for each joint to be injected.

5. A superfical intradermal bleb is to be raised for each injection to eliminate skin sensation.

6. It is important to deliver the fluid accurately in or near the nerve, and this is best assessed by watching the patient's face during the procedure and to injecting at the instant when pain is experienced, as shown by change in facial expression.

7. As a rule, not more than 30ml should be given at each session. This is usually more than adequate, but two sessions may be required in extreme cases.

8. Toxic effects have been minimal in my hands and consist mainly of vertigo, nausea and occasional vasovagal attacks. A cup

of sweet coffee rapidly restores normality. Alternatively, an injection of caffeine.

9. The risk of sepsis is no more than that which occurs with intramuscular injections.

10. Should motor pareses occur, these are only transitory and rarely last for more than two hours. They chiefly occur when treating elbows, resulting in wrist-drop, and occasionally the hips, with transient sciatic nerve paresis.

For success in this treatment one needs only a skin-marking pencil, a 10ml disposable syringe and needle, 0.5% local anaesthetic, Depo-steroid, and a reasonable knowledge of anatomy. The method is devoid of serious complications and when pain has been brought under control, the need for analgesic and anti-inflammatory drugs falls away. It has been found that vitamin supplements are useful in maintaining relief in cases of osteoarthritis, whilst in the treatment of rheumatoid arthritis anti-microorganism drugs should he given concomitantly. [See http:.// www.arthritistrust.org]

These techniques that I have described are suitable for painful joints from any cause provided that the spots I have indicated are tender. It is used mainly in the treatment of Osteoarthritis, but is also used in the treatment of Rheumatoid Arthritis in conjunction with other treatments. Some of the cases of osteoarthritis treated,

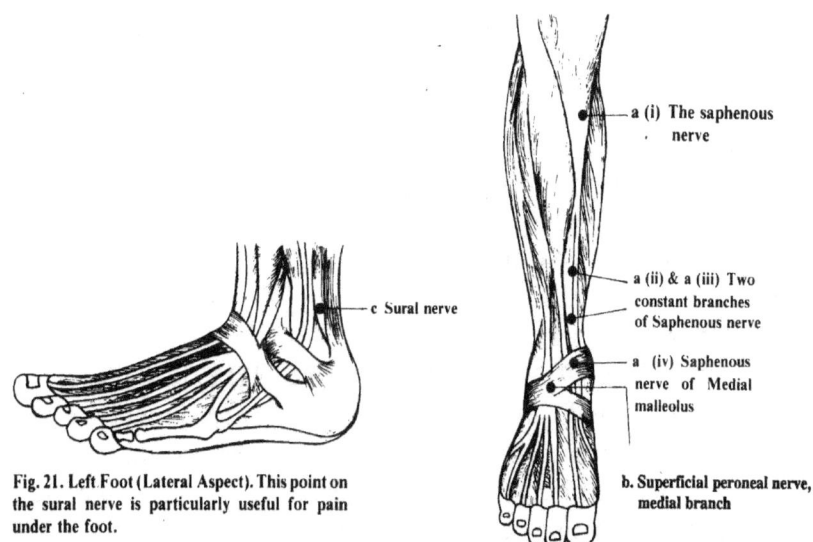

Fig. 21. Left Foot (Lateral Aspect). This point on the sural nerve is particularly useful for pain under the foot.

c Sural nerve

a (i) The saphenous nerve

a (ii) & a (iii) Two constant branches of Saphenous nerve

a (iv) Saphenous nerve of Medial malleolus

b. Superficial peroneal nerve, medial branch

Fig. 20. Right Foot and Leg.

especially in the younger patient and patients with multiple joint infections, can be osteoarthritis lesions secondary to old burnt-out rheumatoid arthritis and in these cases it may be well worth while combining this treatment with that of rheumatoid arthritis, namely the administration of anti-microorganism drugs, particularly of the Imidazole group. [See http://www.arthritistrust.org] This technique is also useful for gout, but likewise this should be treated with anti-gout therapy.

REFERENCES

1. **Gray's Anatomy**. 27th Edition. Longmans Green and Co. London 1938:1104-1105.

2. Pybus PK, *Control of pain and stiffness in the osteoarthritic hand.* S Afr Med J 1981; 59:514.

3. Pybus PK, *A useful physical sign in the painful hand.* S Afr Med .1 1983: 6:598

4. James CDT, Little TF, *Regional hip blockade.* Anaesthesia 1976; 31:l060-1067.

5. Obletz BE, Lockie LM, Mitch E, Hyman 1, *Early effects of partial sensory denervation of the hip for relief of pain in chronic arthritis.* J Bone Joint Surg 1949; 31 A:805.

6. Ergenbright WV, Lowry FC, *Procaine injection for the relief of pain in the hip.* J Bone Joint Surg 1949; 31 A:820.

7. Parkes CR, Kennedy WF, *Obturator nerve block: a simplified approach.* Anaesthesiology 1967; 28:775.

8. Pybus PK, *Osteo-arthrosis of the knee.* Practitioner 1980; 224:928-930.

9. Pybus PK, *Osteoarthritis: a new neurological method of pain control.* Medical Hypotheses 1984; 14(4):413-422.

10. Pybus PK, *Painful flat foot and its management.* S Afr Med J 1981; 59:211.

11. **Grays Anatomy.** 27th Edition. Longmans Green and Co. London 1938:1114.

CHAPTER III
THE MANAGEMENT OF SPONDYLOSIS

The vertebral column is made up of twenty-six individual bones or vertebrae, namely, seven cervical, twelve dorsal or thoracic, five lumbar, and a collection of five sacral vertebrae, which are fused together to constitute one sacral bone. and four coccygeal vertebrae, which are also fused to form the coccyx or tail.

In life each vertebra is attached to the vertebra above and that below by means of various ligaments and an intervertebral fibrocartilaginous disc with a semi-fluid nucleus pulposum, being the endodermal remains of the original foetal spinal column. (Intervertebral joints, one on either side postero lateral to the spinal cord.) The articular surfaces of the two vertebrae display a good deal of gliding action, so that although the whole column is very stable the individual joints are, due to this gliding action, minimally unstable, and with any severe blow or strain on the column, particularly in the cervical area, are easily subluxed. This subluxation is of little threat to the spinal cord, but is a threat to the posterior primary rami as they emerge from the intervertebral foramina and at this point can be compressed.

As a result of this compression non-myelinated fibres are damaged and, in the same way as previously described, the resulting area of nerve damage will act as a generator of abnormal nervous impulses, which in turn will result in the spondylosis or osteoarthritis of the intervertebral joints as described in Chapter I.

A.The Dorsal and Lumbar Spines. These are described first as they are essentially similar, the main nerves involved being the posterior primary rami of T1-T12. They emerge from the intervertebral foramina and run laterally along the transverse process of the vertebra and its pedicle, and it is at this point that the nerve can he safely and easily blocked. Figure 22.

The skin marking is placed over the tenderest spot,which is usually 1.5 to 2cm from the midline between the spinous processes. and the bleb is raised at this place. The needle is then introduced and is directed slightly medially, and if tender spots are encountered on the way, these are injected until the bone is felt, when 2ml of the mixture is instilled.

This is repeated at each tender site found. Figure 23. [Acupuncture nomenclature: Bladder 11-20].

B.The Cervical Spine is the most unstable part of the vertebral column, as the articular facets are hortizontal and flat, whilst further down the column the facets become more vertical and rounded and so stability increases. Thus, in the cervical area subluxation or luxation are relatively common whilst lower down dislocation is rare without a fracture also appearing, and in the lumbar region dislocation without fracture is almost unknown.

The vertebral canal, however, is wide in the cervical region and so subluxation can occur easily without cord damage, but with marked compression of the cervical nerves, which are often involved and damaged by bony projections. This sets up a cervical neuritis with reflex spondylosis.

Space in a booklet such as this does not permit a description of the various syndromes that occur with cervical spondylosis, but it is sufficient to say that if a routine examination of the patient reveals no cause for pain in the neck or headaches, and radiological examination is negative except for the spondylosis, then a routine search for the following tender spots can he made, which if tender should be injected with the mixture as previously described. The points to he palpated are as follows:

1. The Greater Occipital Nerve (Medial Branch of Posterior Primary Ramus of C1)
2. The Lateral Branch of Posterior Primary Ramus Cl
3. The Lesser Occipital Nerve
4. The Greater Auricular Nerve
5. Posterior Primary Rami Cl-C8

1. Greater occipital nerve. The posterior primary ramus of C1 is the largest of the posterior primary rami and emerges from behind the lateral mass of the atlas and inferior to the Occipital artery, then divides into a medial cutaneous and a lateral muscular branch. The medial branch proceeds upwards towards the external occipital protuberance to become the greater occipital nerve and may he found to be tender 1 cm lateral to the protuberance. If tender this is marked, a skin bleb formed, and the needle passed forward and upward to the painful area when 1.5 ml of the mixture is instilled. The injection is very painful and in the more sensitive patients should he done with the subject lying prone. However, with the more stoical it is easier to have the patient sitting with his head flexed. Figure 24(a) [Acupuncture point: Bladder 9].

2. The Lateral branch of posterior primary ramus of C1 is mainly muscular and proceeds downwards as the sub-occipital nerve and supplies the muscles of the sub-occipital triangle. However, a sensory twig from the branch to the inferior oblique muscle joins the posterior primary ramus at C2 and may cause pain and is tender below and lateral to the external protuberance. Figure 24 (h) [Acupuncture point: Bladder 10].

CAUTION: GREAT CARE MUST BE EXERCISED WHEN INJECTING THIS FILAMENT. THE MAIN POSTERIOR PRIMARY RAMUS IS CLOSELY RELATED TO THE VERTEBRAL ARTERY AS IT WINDS ROUND THE LATERAL MASS OF THE ATLAS AND THIS ARTERY IS EASILY DAMAGED OR THE INJECTION MAY BE GIVEN INTRA-ARTERIALLY WITH POSSIBLE EMBARRASSING AND EVEN FATAL RESULTS

It is never necessary to go as deep as the bone, as the filament is compartively superficial; as soon as pain is experienced, only 1 ml of the mixture is injected and with extreme caution. It should not be attempted by the inexperienced.

3. Lesser occipital nerve rises from the anterior primary rami of C2 & 3 and may be found to be tender behind and medial to the mastoid process. It is marked with a skin pencil, a bleb of local is

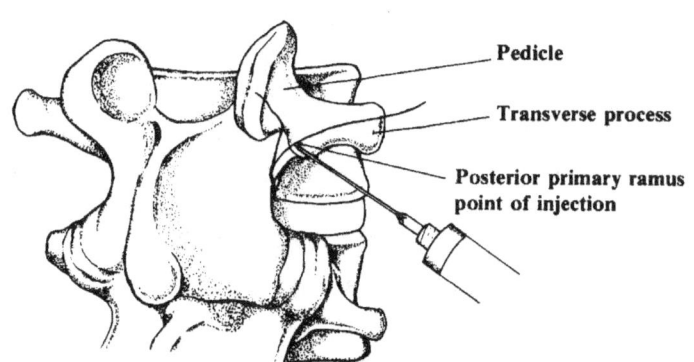

Fig. 22. Postero lateral view of vertebra showing emergence of Posterior primary ramus running upwards over the Pedicle (Medial Branch) and the Transverse process (Lateral Branch). The nerve is usually injected at the bifurcation of the nerve.

raised, and the needle is again directed forward and slightly upward; when pain is felt, 1.2 ml of the mixture is instilled.Figure 24 & 25(c) [Acupuncture point: Gall Bladder 12].

4. Greater auricular nerve C2 & 3. This can be found to be tender at the point where it pierces the deep fascia of the neck, where the external jugular vein crosses the posterior border of the sternomastoid muscle. A bleb is raised over this point and the needle inserted till pain felt and the injection made. Figure 25(d) [Acupuncture point: Small Intestine 16].

5. Third occiptal nerve C2-C8. These are sometimes found 1-2 cm from the midline. Here the needle is introduced through the bleb and passed medially and forwards until bone is felt or pain experienced. One ml of the mixture is usually sufficient. Figure 24(d) [Acupuncture point: nil].

In passing it is to be noted that points 1 and 3 relieve persistent headaches, and that so-called tension headaches are particularly responsive. During the injection, which is often painful, the pain is felt to pass forward to behind the eyes. It lasts however, only a short while, and the headache is immediately relieved.

The greater auricular nerve can he usefully injected in cases of Trigeminal Neuralgia or Tic Doloreux; this technique is described by Wyburn-Mason[1]

It can also be usefully employed for osteoarthritis of the temporomandibular joint and facial palsy[2], amongst others uses.

C. The Lumbosacral Spine. This final subsection is devoted to lesions of the posterior primary rami of L1-S4; it is almost, in effect, the treatment of sciatica or other forms of chronic backache which are usually the precursor of so-called sciatica. The theory was accurately described by Wyburn-Mason, who submitted a thesis on the subject in the fifth decade of this century (1950s) which is reproduced in the original script in Chapter IV and to which this chapter is dedicated.

I will here relate only my own modification of the technique and some of my ideas on the subject. Wyburn-Mason used dehydrated alcohol in his work, aiming at destruction of the posterior primary rami, when the depot steroid was not then available; as the reader will realise, I have substituted my own mixture of local anaesthetic and depot steroid, managing to get results comparable to Wyburn-Mason's. My intention was not to destroy the nerve, but rather to stablise its membrane as I have done elsewhere. However, alcohol can still be employed in obstinate cases but is not recommended for the amateur.

At first it might seem as if this section is diametrically opposed to the belief that cases of sciatica are caused by an intervertebral disc prolapse and that such cases should be treated by laminectomy and removal of the offending disc. However, this is not the case, as both of us point out. There is no doubt that cases showing definite evidence of a prolapsed disc in the L4,5 & S I area, with physical signs of loss of ankle reflex, anaesthesia of the outer side of the calf, and X-ray evidence of a prolapsed disc, should be considered for a laminectomy. However, much of the pain can he caused by nerve entrapment of the posterior primary rami of L1-L3 and Sl-S3 and this can occur as the nerves pierce the fascia lata. Therefore, before submitting a patient with sciatica for laminectomy a search should he made for local tender neuromata and treatment as described elsewhere instituted. If this routine were more widely employed the number of unsuccessful and unnecessary laminectomies would be greatly reduced. In no circumstances should a patient have a repeat laminectomy without this examination being done.

From a study of Figure 26, it will be seen that:

1. The main attack is on the posterior primary rami from L1-L3 and S1-S5.

2. The posterior primary rami of L4 & 5 are small and not in evidence.What there is rapidly anastomoses with the posterior sacral

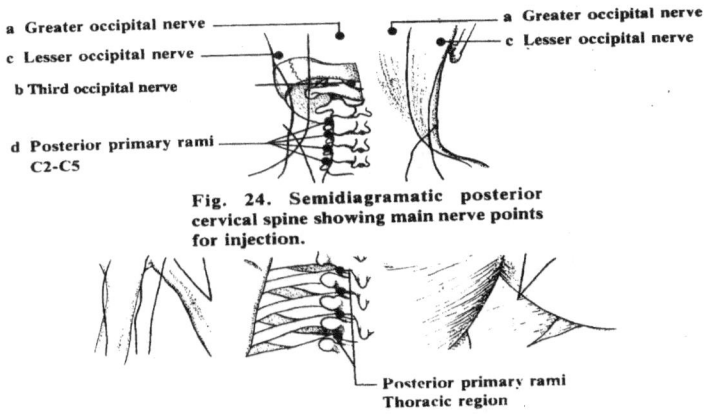

Fig. 24. Semidiagramatic posterior cervical spine showing main nerve points for injection.

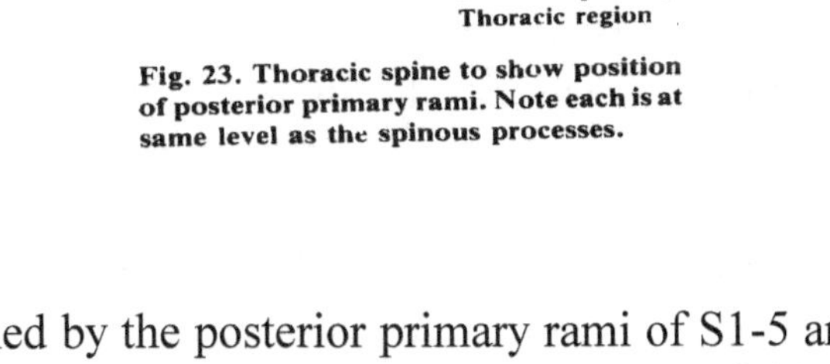

Fig. 23. Thoracic spine to show position of posterior primary rami. Note each is at same level as the spinous processes.

plexus formed by the posterior primary rami of S1-5 and coccygeal nerve. It must be remembered that most successful laminectomies are done for prolapsed disc affecting the L4-5 nerves, the posterior

46

primary rami of which, apart from being very small, would be most inaccessible to injection therapy. For this reason I should wish to stress that intra-neural injection therapy and surgery should not be presented as alternative forms of treatment, but rather the one should complement the other.

I would advocate that the physician should first attempt the intraneural treatment, and if no response is achieved, especially in cases that have physical signs of L4 & 5 nerve involvement, then that patient shall be referred to the neuro-surgeon.

Etiology of sciatic-type pain due to irritation of Posterior Primary Rami.

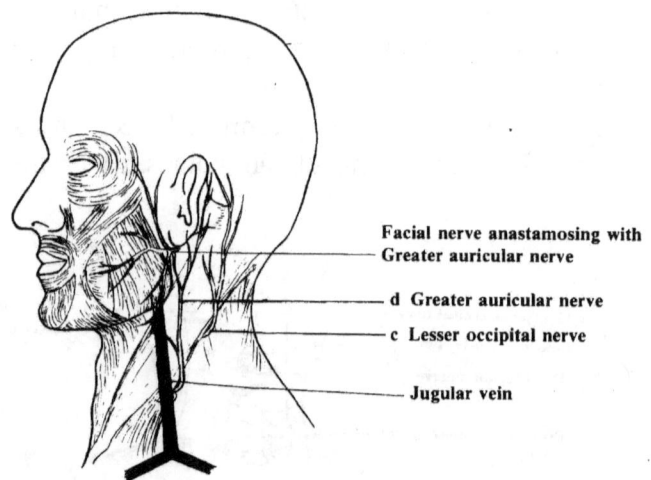

Fig. 25. Head and Neck (Lateral View). The point for injection is where the jugular vein crosses the sternomastoid muscle.

Anatomy.

The fascia lata is attached superiorly to an osteo-ligamentous ring consisting of the sacro-iliac ligament, the back of the sacrum, the sacro-tuberous ligament, the ischium, the inferior ramus of the pubis, the pubic tubercle, the inguinal ligament and the iliac crest. From this upper attachment, the fibres proceed distally and split into two layers into which the insertions of the gluteus maximus and the tensor fascia lata are received. These two muscles are responsible for keeping the fascia tense and for maintaining the upright posture through its lower attachment to the lateral condyle of the tibia and other prominent points round the knee joint. It thus forms a firm tight stocking around the thigh keeping its contents under constant tension. In this tight stocking just below and lateral to the posterior superior iliac spine of the ilium are three rounded lacunae through which the posterior primary rami of the first, second and third sacral nerves are transmitted. In a like manner the three posterior primary rami of the first, second and third lumbar nerves pierce the fascia lata covering the gluteus medius.

Cases of sciatic-type pain commence as a rule with a sacro-iliac strain occurring when the subject is caught off balance, when lifting a heavy weight and from straining from any cause. As a result of this the sacrum rotates slightly in a forward upward and medial direction. This movement causes the tense fascial stocking to be distorted in a longitudinal and lateral direction. This distortion converts the round lacunae into oval slits which compress the nervesproducing trauma. Figure 28.

In 1949 Kelgren[3] showed conclusively that irritation of the posterior primary rami of the areas described produces sciatic-type pain. This he did by injecting 6% hypertonic saline into the nerves, producing sciatica. Furthermore, he found that injecting local anaesthetic into the same nerves relieved the same sciatica that he had created.

Examination

A general examination is essential, especially a rectal examination to exclude any evidence of carcinoma. The neurological investigation should include a search for any loss of sensation in the foot and lower limb, especially on its lateral side, and the presence or absence of the ankle reflex should be noted. The straight-leg-raising test is also done and the angle noted when the pain is first experienced. Fig. 29(a). The patient now lies on his side and a search is made for the following tender points:

i. The Posterior Primary Rami of L 1,2 & 3 are found to he tender in some cases in the upper and inner quadrant of the buttock as they lie in the region below the crest of the ilium. There can be three in number, but usually only two are found. Figure 26c(i).

ii. The Posterior Primary Rami of S1,2 & 3 are nearly always involved and are found on the line of the sacro-iliac joint. Figure 26c(ii). Occasionally that of S4 is also involved, making a total of four points.

48

iii. The coccygeal nerve is occasionally tender to one side of the coccyx and is similarly treated. Figure 26c(iii).

iv. The descending branch of the ilio-hypogastric nerve T12 is also occasionally involved in the process. Figure 26c(iv).

All the above points are treated in the same manner, namely, injection of the mixture through an anaesthetic wheal into the damaged nerve point. The patient is now turned on his back and the straight-leg-raising test repeated. and it will at once be seen how much this has improved. The angle is again noted. Figure 29b.

Discussion

This concept that the tension of the fascia lata causes sciatic-type pain is not new. As far back as 1934 F.R Ober[4] obtained some good results in cases of sciatica by sectioning the ilio-tibial tract. Heyman[5] also described cases of sciatica which had been relieved by stripping the gluteus maximus from its iliac attachment to 'remove pressure on the sciatic nerve'. However, it is not difficult to imagine that in doing this he probably sectioned the Posterior Primary Rani of S1,2 & 3, so producing a cure.

REFERENCES

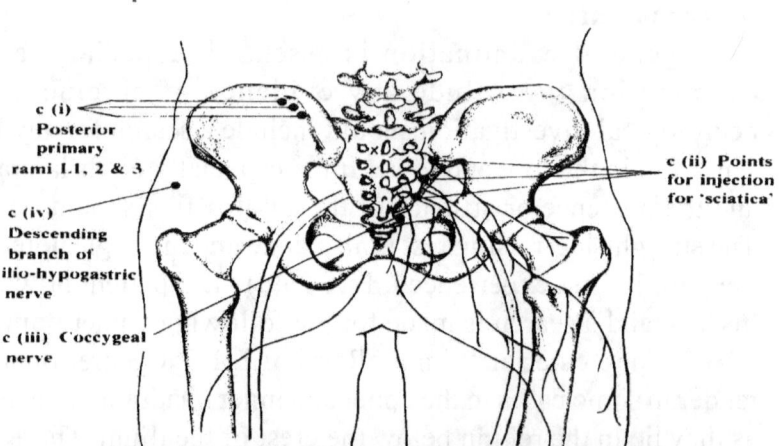

c (i)
Posterior
primary
rami 1.1, 2 & 3

c (iv)
Descending
branch of
ilio-hypogastric
nerve

c (iii) Coccygeal
nerve

c (ii) Points
for injection
for 'sciatica'

Fig. 26. Posterior view of Pelvis showing the Sciatic nerve and the posterior primary rami of S1-4 forming the posterior sacral plexus. The three most commonly used points are marked with a solid black circle on the right. Other useful points shown by X on the left side.

1. Wyburn-Mason R, *The Nature of Tic Doloreaux* . Brit. Med. J. July 18, 1953. pp. 119-122

2. Wyburn-Mason R, *The Nature of Bell's Palsy.* Brit. Med. .1. Sept. 18, 1954, pp. 679-681

3. Kellgren J H, *Deep Pain Sensibility.* Lancet 1947; 1:943

4.Ober FR, *Back Strain & Sciatica.* J.A.M.A. 1935; 104:1580

5. Heyman CH, *Thoughts on Relief of Sciatic Pain.* J. Bone & Joint Surgery. 1947; 73: 355.

CHAPTER IV
IS 'SCIATICA' A LESION OF THE SCIATIC NERVE OR ITS COMPONENTS?
TREATMENT OF SCIATICA BY ALCOHOL INJECTIONS INTO THE BUTTOCK

by

R. Wyburn-Mason, M.A., M.D. (Camb.)

INTRODUCTION

This chapter, written by Roger Wyburn-Mason, but never, as far as I am aware, ever actually published, is included here out of respect for this great man to whom I had the honour to be House Physician in 1951.

The principles involved are the same as I now use in treating arthritic joints by intra-neural injections. This is an idea originated by Wyburn-Mason and modified and developed by myself. It has stood me in good stead with my many patients, the great majority of whom have got endless relief of pain and stiffness.

Sciatica, as its name implies, was thought for many years to be due to disturbance of function, possibly inflammatory in nature, in the sciatic nerve (see Wilson, 1940)[3]. However, it is uncommon to find any pathological changes in the nerve on the rare opportunities when microscopical examination has been possible; although occasionally such changes have been reported (Wiedel and LeSourd, 1902[2] Hunt, 1905[3]; Denny-Brown 1933[4]. In other cases arthritis of the hip, congenital anomalies of the fifth lumbar and first sacral vertebrae or lesions of the sacroiliac joint are thought to be the basis of the symptoms. According to Wilson, "fibrositis -- lumbar or gluteal -- is another outstanding cause, not perhaps rigidly separable" from sciatic neuritis (see Yawgcr, 1911[5]; Helweg, 1920[6]; Petre'n, 1921[7]; Linstedt, 1921[8] Jansen, 1921[9]).

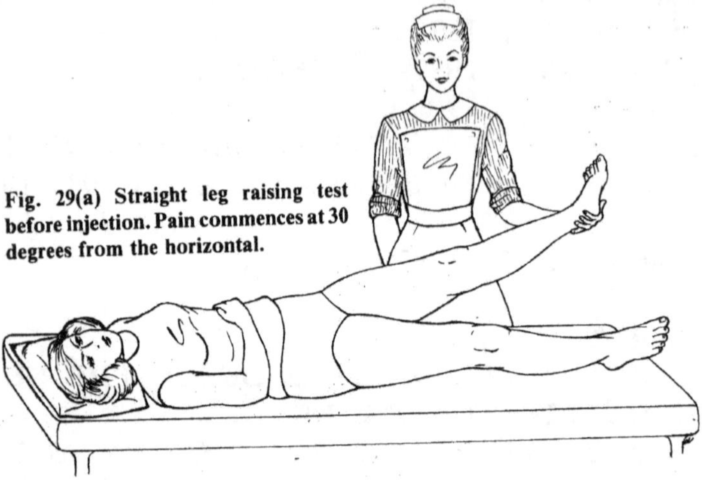

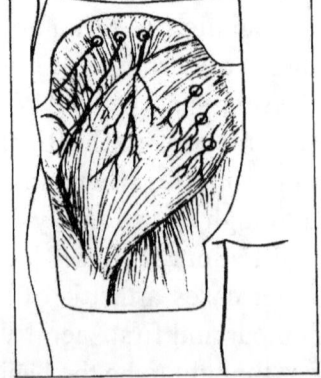

50

Fig. 29(a) Straight leg raising test before injection. Pain commences at 30 degrees from the horizontal.

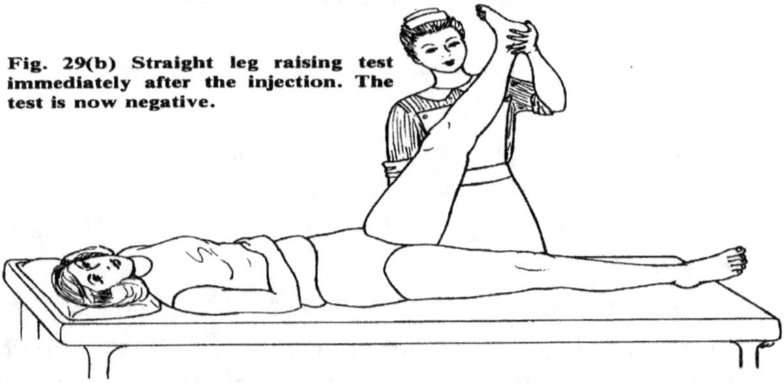

Fig. 29(b) Straight leg raising test immediately after the injection. The test is now negative.

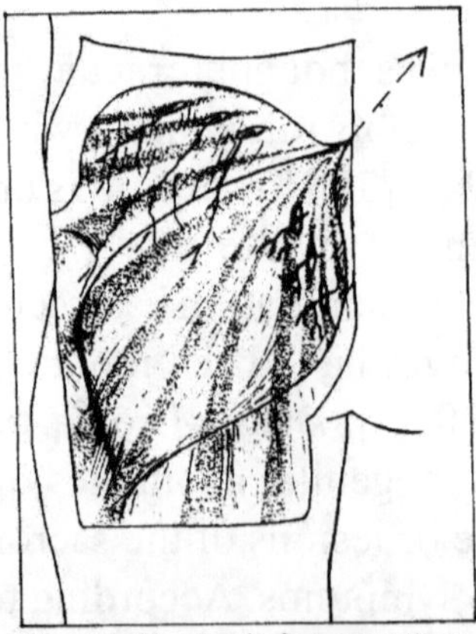

Fig. 28. The fascia is now put on the stretch due to the movement of the posterior superior iliac spine. The now oval lucanae are shown pinching the nerves. The lines of force are clearly shown.

Fig. 27. The fascia lata semidigramatic showing the posterior primary rami perforating through round lacunae.

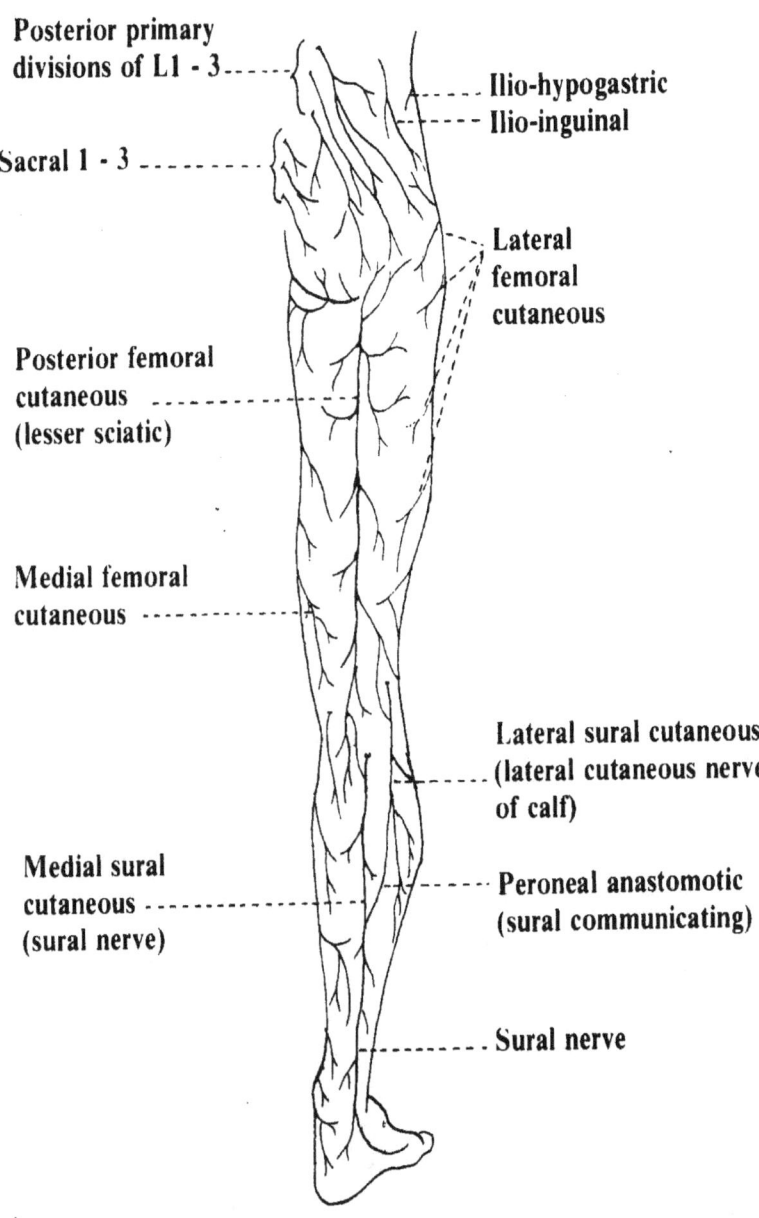

Posterior primary
divisions of L1 - 3

Ilio-hypogastric
Ilio-inguinal

Sacral 1 - 3

Lateral
femoral
cutaneous

Posterior femoral
cutaneous
(lesser sciatic)

Medial femoral
cutaneous

Lateral sural cutaneous
(lateral cutaneous nerve
of calf)

Medial sural
cutaneous
(sural nerve)

Peroneal anastomotic
(sural communicating)

Sural nerve

Figure 30   The cutaneous nerves of the right lower extremity and buttock. Note the fact that the distal branches of the lateral and posterior femoral cutaneous nerves ramify and join with the origin of the lateral and medial sural cutaneous nerves near the head of the fibula.

Sciatica may also occur as a so-called reflex lesion during and after pregnancy and in association with renal calculi. In the last 20 years, however, through the discovery of the importance of the diseased intervertebral disc, in some quarters opinion has swung to the belief that almost all cases of sciatica are due to rupture or herniation of the nucleus pulposus of the disc between L4 and 5 or L5 and S1 vertebrae, and operations designed to remove pressure on the affected nerve roots have been undertaken enthusiastically. In the opinion of many, however, since the majority of cases improve without operation, such interference is unjustifiable. In addition, at operation it is common to find no obvious distributions. Pain of the first type occurred more often than the second in the ratio of 2.3 to 1. It is often accompanied by a burning sensation and occasionally by paraesthesiae, which are especially liable to affect or are often confined to the outer and lower aspect of the calf. Sometimes they involve the dorsum of the foot, big toes or lateral border of the foot. In a small proportion of cases (about 1 in 10 of my series), pain may be felt in the groin or perineum especially on coughing or straining.

Sensory impairment is rare and, if present at all, is slight and confined to the lower and outer part of the calf and occasionally to the outer border or dorsum of the foot. The skin of the buttock may be sensitive and the patient dislike sitting, which causes the skin of the buttock to become numb. The pain is either eased or made worse by movement or by resting and may become severe and sharp in the lumbar or gluteal region or leg on coughing, sneezing or bending. It is increased by flexion of the hip with the knee straight (Lasegue's sign) and by flexion of the spine (Kernig's sign). Only very infrequently is there any muscular weakness and it is then confined to slight foot-drop.

Other muscles are unaffected and there is rarely much muscular wasting. The ankle jerk may be exaggerated, normal or diminished. There may, however, be a loss of tone of the buttock, hamstrings, calf and leg muscles. The gluteal fold, which results from fascial tension and adherence to subcutaneous fat is often diminished or lost, presumably as a result of some local trophic change[1] (Wilson, 1940). As already mentioned, sacral, lumbar or gluteal points of tenderness (fibrositis) have frequently been found and many have laid stress on their presence in the gluteal region in cases of sciatica.

There is said to be tenderness on pressure at the sacro-sciatic notch, gluteal fold, middle of the back of the thigh, back of the knee, below the head of the fibula or behind the lateral malleolus (Valleix's points). However, in the writer's experience these are by no means constantly present. In my series of cases of sciatica, I found that there is in about 70% of subjects acute tenderness on pressure in one of two regions. In cases in which the pain occurs in the lateral part of the buttock and thigh these points are in the upper and outer quadrant of the buttock and I have called them the lateral gluteal points.* (*P.P.R. of L,1-3 P.K.P. see Chapter III) Pressure here results in marked pain both locally and often spreading down the leg in the distribution of the spontaneous pain. It may also give rise to paraesthesiae in the lower and outer side of the calf. In these cases there is rarely tenderness over the sacro-sciatic notch or back of the thigh (Valleix's points). On the other hand, in cases where spontaneous pain is in the posterior part of the buttock and thigh there is often severe tenderness on pressure in the medial part of the upper gluteal region, the medial gluteal points **. (**P.P.R. of S1-3 P.K.P. see Chapter III) Pressure here causes both local pain and radiation to the regions where spontaneous pain occurs. i.e., down the back of the thigh and outer side of the calf.

Only in these cases did I find tenderness over the Valleix's points in the middle of the back of the thigh and gluteal fold and near the sacro-sciatic notch. It is usually considered that in cases of sciatica pain is elicited from pressure over the sciatic nerve at the notch, but this does not seem to be so, as the tender spots are just medial to the lateral border of the sacrum and extend considerably above the notch. Occasionally there is tenderness over both the "lateral" and "medial gluteal points". In both types of case tender Valleix's points below the head of the fibula and behind the lateral malleolus may be present.

It is to be observed that the skin of the buttock is painful, may tingle and feel numb and shows trophic changes. The deep tissues of the upper part of the buttock are also painful and tender. The pain may also extend to the groin and to the perineum occasionally. None of these tissues are supplied by the sciatic nerve. The flexor muscles of the hip joint and the flexor and extensor muscles of the lumbar spine and the psoas muscle and sphincter ani are in spasm and are innervated by L1-4 & S2-4 nerve roots rather than by those contributing to the sciatic nerve.

The effects of local anaesthesia or alcohol injection into the buttock in cases of sciatica.

Cases of 'sciatica' conforming to the above description have been treated first by local anaesthetic and afterwards by absolute alcohol injection into the tender lateral or medial gluteal points. The tender spots, which number 3-8 or more, are found by deep pressure and marked with a skin pencil. The skin is then anaesthetized with 2 percent procaine or lignocaine and a long needle is passed through the skin till it touches the bone. Two mls. of anaesthetic are infiltrated, the needle withdrawn slightly and directed at various angles and various depths, and further anaesthetic injected. This almost without exception results in complete relief of all pain and paraesthesiae both above and below the level of the injection for the duration of the anaesthesia.

This effect is mentioned by Brain[10] (1951). The relief is, however, usually only temporary and the pain returns when the effect of the anaesthetic wears off. It was, therefore, decided to inject alcohol. Five to ten mls. of absolute alcohol infiltrated into the gluteal muscle at different depths and directions from 1/4 inch (0.6 cms.) away from the bone to within an inch (2.5 cms.) of the skin surface, care being taken not to inject the alcohol into the skin for fear of causing necrosis. As much as 40 mls. may be given without ill-effects. *Great care must he taken not to inject in the neighborhood of the sciatic nerve.* The injection of alcohol causes transient severe pain both locally and passing upwards and down the lower limb in the distribution of the spontaneous pain. When the lateral gluteal points are injected the pain goes down the lateral aspect of the hip and thigh and calf to the foot; when the medial points, it extends down the posterior aspect of the thigh. Either may be accompanied by paraesthesiae in the calf and foot. The pain lasts only 1-2 minutes and is followed by some local aching for 30 minutes or so and by stiffness in the buttock for some days.

Some 167 cases of "sciatica" with the above characteristics as of duration varying from 10 weeks to several years have been treated. All these had failed to respond to previous treatment by rest, radiant heat, massage, analgesics, etc. Those which exhibited abnormal features either in the distribution of the pain or paraesthesiae or by loss of the knee jerk were not included. In about half the cases (77), when the pain of the injection died down, the patient volunteered dramatic immediate relief of symptoms in the leg and in about 3 days there was almost complete relief of symptoms in the buttock also. In the other half, while there was immediately considerable diminution in intensity, some pain persisted, generally only in the calf and foot as well as a certain amount of ache at the site of the injection. If the pain was present after two weeks, it was usually found that some tender points remained in the buttock and these were re-injected. This was necessary in 52 cases. In only 19 cases, usually patients with very fat buttocks, was a third injection required. In 7 cases some slight lower leg and foot pain persisted in spite of treatment and in 12 the pain was only partly relieved.

Unexpectedly, when successful, the injection usually rapidly abolished the lumbar pain and muscle spasm as well as that in the buttock, thigh and leg. In cases in which the ankle jerk was lost this usually returned in the course of 4-12 weeks. The injection gave no relief of symptoms in cases of sciatica in which the pain did not extend into the upper gluteal region and where no tenderness was present there. A typical example of successful treatment was the following:

Case I. Male, age 46. Gardener. Four years previously he had suffered from acute lumbago, the symptoms lasting for 3-4 weeks. This recurred several times in the next 4 years, the attacks being precipitated by exposure to damp or bending down at his work. In all the attacks pain had extended from the mid-lumbar region to the upper and outer quadrant of the buttock. Radio-graphs of his lumbar spine had been taken and proved normal. Three months prior to hospital attendance he had another attack and, in spite of rest and rubbing with ointments prescribed by his doctor, pain persisted. In fact, after a particularly prolonged massage of the lumbar region and buttock the pain rapidly spread down the outer side of the right hip and thigh to the outer-side of the calf and ankle. It had remained very severe, was agonizing on coughing and was accompanied by a numb, tingling sensation in the outer side of the right calf. Coughing caused sharp pains in the buttock extending to the groin and perineum. After 2 months he noticed that his foot tended to flop when walking. He had been unable to work for 3 months.

Examination. Lumbar muscle spasm severe, especially on the right with loss of lordosis, producing a scoliosis with convexity to the left. All movements of the lumbar spine restricted. Unable to put his right heel on the ground because it caused pain. Acutely tender over the right lateral gluteal points, pressure here causing pain down the leg and tingling in the calf. Loss of the gluteal fold on the right. Lase'gue's sign positive at 25 degrees on the right and 60 degrees on the left. Right ankle jerk unobtainable, left ankle and both knee jerks normal. Plantar responses flexor. Some blunting of sensation to pin-prick, but not to other modalities, in the skin on the outer side of the calf. Some weakness of the right anterior tibial muscles. Muscle electrical responses were normal. Radiographs of the lumbar and sacral spine normal, apart from scoliosis and loss of lordosis. C.S.F., normal, protein 40mgms.%., 4 lymphocytes per cu. mm.

The lateral gluteal points were injected with alcohol as described, a total of 25 mls being used. This caused severe pain in the distribution of the spontaneous pain and tingling in the outer side of the calf. Half an hour later the patient volunteered that the pain in the leg had ceased. There was still some lumbar aching and also aching in the region of the injection. He was sent to rest at home. One week later he still complained of some lumbar pain, slight aching in the region of the injection and in the calf only on walking. He was able to sleep at night and required 2 aspirin tablets only occasionally. Examination now showed marked diminution in the lumbar muscle spasm and scoliosis. The muscle weakness was not detectable, though the ankle jerk was still unobtainable. Sensory loss now indefinite. He was still tender over a number of points in the upper and outer quadrant of the buttock. These were re-injected with alcohol (a total of 10 mls). He was seen 10 days later, when he stated that his only symptom was some aching in the lumbar region after standing. The scoliosis, loss of lumbar lordosis and muscle spasm had disappeared. The ankle jerk was still unobtainable. He returned to work a week later. Three months after the first injection the ankle jerk returned.

Sciatica arising from lesions high in the buttock.

Occasionally lesions high in the musculature of the buttock give rise to typical sciatica. This is exemplified by the following:

Case 2. A soldier, aged 22, sustained a shrapnel wound of the muscle of the upper and outer quadrant of the right buttock. The metal was removed a few hours later and the wound healed rapidly. but some days afterwards he developed pain in the region of the wound passing down the back and posterolateral aspect of the thigh to the outer side of the calf, outer malleolus and dorsum of the foot and upwards into the lumbar region. It had persisted with varying severity for some 3 years, When examined at the end of this time, he was found to be tender on deep pressure at several spots in the upper and outer quadrant of the buttock near the wound. Lase'gue's sign was positive on this side. There was loss of lumbar lordosis with lumbar muscle spasm. The ankle jerk was lost. Radiographs of the lumbo-sacral spine were normal. On two occasions the tender areas were injected with alcohol as described above. The first caused a severe but short-lived exacerbation of pain in the distribution of that occurring spontaneously. Afterwards he complained of a floppiness of his foot and, when examined, there was a mild weakness of the dorsiflexors of the ankle and toes. After a second injection he was completely relieved of all sensory symptoms, except for an occasional local aching at the injection site. The muscle weakness disappeared in a fortnight and the ankle jerk had returned two months later.

On intramuscular injection of substances which cause pain, such as penicillin, into the upper and outer quadrant of the buttock the pain tends to radiate down the outer side of the thigh and calf and even into the foot, as the writer himself has experienced. In certain circumstances it may give rise to a typical attack of sciatica. This was observed in the following case:

Case 3. A female patient of 63 years suffering from congestive heart failure was receiving twice weekly injections of mersalyl intramuscularly into the upper and outer quadrant of the buttock. Two weeks after beginning treatment, immediately after one of these injections, she developed severe pain identical in distribution and character with that in the last case. She was found to be acutely tender in the same place (at the site of the injection). Lase'gue's sign was positive. Her symptoms dramatically disappeared after a single injection of 5 mls of alcohol into the tender spots in the buttock. Intramuscular injections of substances, e.g. bismuth, into the buttock as a cause of sciatica are also mentioned by Grinker and Bucy (1949)[11].

The effects of local anaesthetization of the lateral
or posterior femoral cutaneous nerves in cases of sciatica.

As already described, in the thigh the site of the pain in cases of sciatica is either on the lateral or posterior aspect, apparently in the area of distribution of the lateral or posterior femoral cutaneous nerves respectively. The effect of anaesthetization of these nerves by infiltration with 2% lignocaine solution was examined in eight cases, four with pain in the lateral and four in the posterior distribution. The lateral femoral cutaneous nerve is palpated a little medial to the anterior superior iliac spine as it emerges from beneath the inguinal ligament and located by the tenderness on pressure. The posterior femoral cutaneous nerve is found as it emerges from beneath the gluteus maximus muscle in the mid-line of the back and thigh. In order to avoid the sciatic nerve during anaesthetization, the needle is not inserted into the muscle beneath the nerve. About 5 ccs. of anaesthetic were injected into each location. The sciatic nerve was unaffected, as no motor weakness or sensory loss in the sciatic distribution was induced. It was found that when the pain was in the lateral distribution, anaesthetization of the lateral femoral cutaneous nerve abolished much of it below the site of injection. When the posterior nerve was also injected practically all pain below the site of injection was relieved. When the pain was chiefly in the posterior part of the thigh, almost all the pain was relieved by block of the posterior femoral cutaneous nerve.

Comparison of the symptoms of sciatica with those of lesions of the sciatic nerve.

It is of interest to compare the condition of sciatica with the known effects of disturbance of the sciatic nerve or of its constituent roots. An irritative lesion, such as a gun-shot wound of the great sciatic nerve high in the thigh, gives rise to causalgia. This causes excruciating pain which is felt in the sole of the foot, in the plantar surface of the toes and also, perhaps, in the calf, but not in the buttock or lumbar region. The sole becomes lengthened, narrowed and oval rather than cuboid with longitudinal folds or furrows in the skin. The foot may also be oedematous; the nail structure becomes altered and the skin is mottled, hot and hyperaemic or is markedly cold and sweating. Total paralysis of the sciatic nerve results in loss of the power of flexion at knee, ankle and toes, of extension of ankle and toes and of in- and eversion of the foot. The corresponding muscles waste and there is a loss of sensation in the outer surface of the calf, instep, sole of foot and toes, only the inner side of the leg and ankle escaping. The ankle jerk is lost.

Incomplete lesions tend to affect the peroneal (lateral popliteal) division more commonly, giving rise to paralysis of the peronei, tibialis anterior and toe extensors and eventually leading to pied-en-griffe. Sensation is lost over the outer side and lower third of the anterior aspect of the leg, on the instep and in the dorsal surface of the four inner toes at their proximal end. There may be some swelling of the foot, local cyanosis and coldness, anhidrosis and thinning of the skin over the dorsum with increased thickness of the sole. The ankle jerk is preserved. Involvement of the tibial (medial popliteal) nerve causes paralysis of the calf muscles and foot flexors and weakness of inversion of the foot. The small muscles of the foot atrophy and tend to cause claw-foot. Loss of sensation is found over the sole and heel, lower third of the posterior aspect of the leg, plantar surface of the toes and dorsum of the terminal phalanges with loss of the ankle jerk.

This clinical picture is completely different from that occuring in ordinary cases of sciatica in the distribution of the pain, sensory disturbance, motor weakness and the occurrence of severe trophic changes in the former, but not in the latter. In cases of sciatic nerve lesions there is no lumbar, psoas or anal sphincter muscle spasm, no pain or sensory disturbance in the buttock, groin and perineum and no trophic lesions in the buttock as in cases of sciatica.

CONCLUSIONS

It seems that 1) the symptoms of sciatica are different from those resulting from an irritative lesion of the sciatic nerve and its constituent roots, 2) in a large proportion of cases of sciatica there is severe tenderness on pressure over the upper gluteal musculature, 3) painful injections or lesions in the upper gluteal musculature lead to aching pain similar in nature and distribution to that occuring in cases of sciatica, 4) the symptoms of sciatica are relieved by local anaesthetization or alcohol injections into certain tender areas deep in the upper part of the gluteal muscles at the sites where the muscles take origin from the iliac bone, and 5) the nervous pathway of the pain impulses in the thigh is the lateral and/or posterior femoral cutaneous nerves. This suggests that the primary disturbance in many cases of sciatica is a lesion in this part of the gluteal muscles, possibly of the aponeurotic origin of the gluteal muscles from the ilium, a lesion perhaps induced by excessive muscle use or muscle tearing as in lifting heavy weights or bending.

Lase'gue's or Kernig's manoeuvers may give rise to pain, not because they stretch the sciatic nerve, but rather the gluteal muscles.

What is the mechanism by which a lesion of the origins of the gluteal muscles from the ilium causes sciatic pain in the lower limbs and in the lumbar region, spasm of the lumbar, psoas and sphincter ani muscles and occasionally footdrop and loss of the ankle jerk? Kellgren (1929)[12]. investigated the reference of pain arising when hypertonic saline solutions were injected into various deep structures, such as interspinous ligaments, periostea, aponeuroses, etc. Pain is referred to other branches of the nerve or nerve roots supplying the structures concerned. It is necessary to consider the sensory nerve supply of the gluteal region to understand the phenomena of sciatica.

The skin, subcutaneous tissue and muscles of the gluteal region receive their sensory innervation from four directions, superiorly, laterally, medially and inferiorly. a) Superiorly, the lateral branches of the posterior primary divisions of the upper three lumbar nerve roots pierce the fleshy part of the ilio-costalis muscle and the aponeurosis of the latissimus dorsi, cross the iliac crest near the edge of the erector spinae muscle or pass through the lumbar (Petit's) triangle and terminate in the subcutaneous tissue and skin and the gluteal muscle of the outer part of the gluteal region (see Fig. 3(a)). Filaments pass down as far as the greater trochanter of the femur and even lower. These nerves constitute the *nervii clunium superiores.* b) Laterally, branches of the ilio-inguinal nerves formed from the anterior primary divisions of L1 nerve root, and the posterior branches of the lateral femoral cutaneous nerves formed from the anterior primary divisions of L2-3 roots pass back to supply both the skin and gluteal muscles. c) Medially, the lateral branches of the posterior primary divisions of the fifth lumbar nerve roots pass downwards to join the lateral branches of the first sacral posterior primary division. The posterior divisions of the sacral nerve roots, except the last, issue from the posterior foramina of the sacrum. The first three are covered at their exit from the bone by the multifidus muscle and, like other posterior primary divisions, immediately bifurcate. The lateral branches of S1-3 join with one another and with those of L5 and S4 to form a series of anastomoses on the upper part of the sacrum, the *posterior sacral plexus*. From these, branches are directed upwards to the posterior surface of the great sacro-sciatic ligament, where they are covered by the gluteus maximus muscle and form a second series of loops to end as cutaneous nerves, the *nervi clunium mediales*. These latter pierce the gluteus maximus to pass outwards over the muscle. d) Inferiorly, the posterior femoral cutaneous nerve (small or lesser sciatic) arises from the dorsal branches of the anterior rami of S2 and 3 nerve roots. After leaving the pelvis and reaching the lower border of gluteus maximus, it gives off 3 or 4 gluteal branches (*nervi clunium inferniores*), which turn upwards round the lower border of gluteus maximus. They supply the skin over the lower and lateral part of the muscle and anastomose with the branches of the nervi clunium mediales and superiores and the branches of the ilio-inguinal and lateral femoral cutaneous nerves to form the *cluneal plexus*, lying subcutaneously and in the muscles.

In cases of sciatica the whole of the buttock is very sore and sensitive, readily becomes numb and shows trophic changes. This suggests that the cluneal plexus is irritated. From the gluteal region the pain of sciatica extends in the distribution of the posterior femoral cutaneous nerve from S2-3 roots (back of thigh and calf), of the ilio-inguinal and lateral femoral cutaneous nerves L1-3 (lateral side of hip thigh and groin), of the sacral nerve roots (perineum) and into the lumbar region (lumbar nerve roots). All these areas are supplied by sensory nerves which also contribute fibres to the cluneal plexus. The muscles in spasm are those of the lumbar spine (flexors, extensors and rotators) and psoas. all of which are innervated from L1-4 nerve roots, and the sphincter ani muscle, innervated by S2-4 nerve roots, all of which roots also contribute fibres to the cluneal plexus. Thus, the muscle spasm and most of the pain in cases of sciatica are readily explicable as referred along the branches and roots of the nerves contributing to the irritated cluneal plexus.

How do pain, paraesthesiae and motor weakness appear below the knee? The posterior femoral cutaneous nerve runs down the back of the thigh superficial to the long head of the biceps and beneath the fascia. It supplies the skin and subcutaneous tissues at the back of the thigh and in the poplitcal space (see Fig. 1). At the back of the knee it pierces the deep fascia and passes down as far as the middle of the calf of the leg, its terminal twig joining the sural nerve. This latter is formed of the medial sural cutaneous branch (sural nerve), of the tibial (medial popliteal) nerve and the peroneal anastomotic (sural communicating) branch of the common peroneal (lateral popliteal). The sural nerve passes down the outer side of the calf to the region behind the lateral malleolus and then forwards below the malleolus to the lateral side of the foot and little toes, communicating on the dorsum of the foot with the superficial peroneal branch of the common peroneal nerve. Branches of the lateral cutaneous nerve pass down and innervate the skin and superficial tissues on the outside of the thigh and knee reaching as far as the head of the fibula. In this region originates the superficial peroneal (musculo-cutaneous) and medial (sural communicating) and lateral sural cutaneous (lateral cutaneous nerve of calf) branches of the common peroneal nerve, with branches of which the finer filaments of the lateral femoral cutaneous nerve join. The superficial peroneal nerve winds subcutaneously round the head of the fibula and supplies the peronei muscles. This nerve divides into medial and intermediate dorsal cutaneous nerves above the ankle. The former passes to supply the medial side of the great toe and adjacent sides of the second and third toes, the latter the adjacent side of the third, fourth and fifth toes and the skin on the lateral side of the ankle, communicating with the sural nerve. Often lateral branches of the superficial peroneal nerve are absent and their function is taken over by the sural nerve. Nerve fibres, in fact, usually reach the skin of the dorsum of the foot and toes partly in the branches of the superficial peroneal and partly by way of the lateral sural cutaneous branch of the same common peroneal nerve and thence via the peroneal anastomotic nerve and sural nerve to the dorsum of the foot. In some cases only the latter route is taken. When motor weakness appears in cases of sciatica, it is always in the muscles innervated by the superficial peroneal nerve, paralysis of which causes foot-drop. When pain and sensory loss exist below the knee, they are found a) in the lower one-third of the outer side of the calf, which is innervated by the lateral sural nerves, and/or b) on the outer side of the ankle and foot, and/or c) in the dorsum of the foot (both of which latter areas may be innervated solely through the sural nerve or partly through its branches and those of the superficial peroneal nerve). Thus, the motor and sensory loss below the knee in cases of 'sciatica' must be due to disturbance of fibres on the superficial peroneal, lateral sural cutaneous and sural nerves. Now, the terminal twigs of the lateral or posterior femoral nerves, irritated in cases of sciatica, join the superficial peroneal and lateral sural cutaneous nerves as they lie very superficially in the region of the head of the fibula, and branches of the posteior femoral cutaneous actually join the sural nerve. Thus, it may be that the motor weakness and sensory disturbance below the knee are produced by the reflex irritation of the posterior and lateral femoral cutaneous nerves extending into the superficial peroneal, sural or lateral sural cutaneous nerves. So, the variable sensory and motor loss found in cases of sciatica could be explained.

SUMMARY

Clinical and experimental evidence is adduced to show that in many cases of sciatica the symptoms are the result not of a lesion of the sciatic nerve or of its component nerve roots, but of a disturbance of the gluteal muscles high in the buttock which results in an irritation of the cluneal nerve plexus and the reference of pain in various directions.

A method of treating cases by alcohol injection into the buttock is described.

REFERENCES

1 . Brain W R, (1951). **Diseases of the Nervous System**. 4th Edit. Oxford Medical Publications, London.

2. Denny-Brown DE, (1933) Proc. R. Soc. Med., 26 1399.

3. Grinker, RR & Bucy, PS (1949). **Neurology.** Blackwell, Oxford.

4. Helweg J, (1920) **Ischias.** Thesis. Copenhagen.

5. Hunt J, (1905) Amer. Med., 9, 620.

6. Jansen H, (1921) Lancet. ii. 737.

7. Kellgren J H, (1939). Clin. Sci. 4. 35.

8. Lindstedt F, (1921). Acta. Med. Scand. 55. 248.

9. Petren K, (1921). Acta. Med. Scand, 55. 229.

10. Wiedel, F & i.e. Sourd, L (1902). Bull. Mem. Soc. Med. Hop. Paris, 19. 1046.

11. Wilson SAK, (1940) **Neurology.** Arnold. London.

12.Yawger NS, (1911) Boston Med. Surg. J. 164. 843.

CHAPTER V
OSTEOARTHRITIS OF THE HIP AND OTHER POINTS

Treatment of osteoarthritis of the hip is today usually by means of joint replacement and the results of this operation are as a rule very good now that the mechanics of the operation are better understood.

The operation has, however, some drawbacks, namely:

1. The operation has to be performed by a surgeon versed in its execution and with a good record.

2. Expense can he enormous.

3. Sepsis is a disaster and should it occur can produce dire terminal results.

4. Loss of proprioception in joint cavity.

5. Rejection of prosthesis produces girdlestone condition.

6. The patient can't spare the time involved.

7. The head of the femur is now an inanimate object and can only wear out.

As you all know, I have, thanks to the motivation given to me by Roger Wyburn-Mason, developed a method of controlling pain and stiffness in all rheumatoid joints which I have described to you in the past and this has also been taken up by Gus Prosch, Jr., M.D., and now also many other physicians.

The broad principles of these neural blocks is that the disease is not primarily in the joint cavity, but rather in the peripheral nerve that has been damaged. This damaged nerve gives off ectopic nerve impulses in both directions, both prodromic that produces spasm and antidromic which gives rise to peripheral inflammation. These two give all the symptoms and signs of osteoarthritis of every joint and the hip is no exception.

The main nerves involved in the process are:

1. **The obturatur nerve** which enters the thigh through the obturatur fora-men and divides into an anterior and posterior branch and terminates along the medial side of the femur, approximately 20 centimetres below the anterior superior iliac spine of the pelvis. It gives a branch to the hip joint on its anterior surface and other muscular branches to adductors of the hip. These points exist where they can be tender due to neural damage. They are:

a. as it enters the thigh in the groin;

b. as it terminates 20 centimetres on the medial side of the femur:

c. over its articular branch on the anterior surface of the joint. If tender, these spots require injections.

2. **The lateral femoral cutaneous nerve** which enters the thigh below and medial to the anterior superior iliac spine to supply the skin over the lateral side of the thigh. It is severely tender in practically all cases and especially those of fixed flexion. Injection

of this nerve abolishes most cases of fixed flexion as is determined by Thomas's Test.

3. **The femoral nerve** gives off a branch to the rectus femoris muscle which in turn gives an articular branch to the upper surface of the hip joint. It is the latter that is found tender over the superior aspect of the greater trochanter. A further branch is also given off in the groin anterior to the femoral vessels and this branch occasionally when tender requires injection.

4. **The nerve to quadratus femoris** enters the thigh anterior or deep to the sciatic nerve; as well as supplying the muscle it gives off branches to the posterior surface of the hip joint. These may be two or three in number and may require separate injections.

The above will show the complete absence of the sciatic nerve involvement which takes no part in the process whatsoever.

Procedure

1. The patient lies on his back on the couch and all the movements of the joint are examined and the degree of fixed flexion noted.

The thigh is now palpated in front and tender spots may he found in the groin, below and medial to anterior superior iliac spine or over the medial side of the thigh. These points are all injected to increase the abduction removing adductor spasm and also by abolishing fixed flexion.

The patient is now turned onto his side and the greater trochanter is carefully palpated. Three spots are often found, namely, anterior, superior and posterior to the trochanter. Blebs are raised one centimetre peripherally to the spots and a long needle introduced in a centregrade fashion to enter the nerve under the shelf of the trochanteric ridge. These are all injected with the result of increased and painless mobility of the joints.

Results

The patient is told that this treatment, although appearing miraculous at the time, in point of fact often requires repeated sessions of injections, although each injection is less severe than the last. I usually suggest that they have at least three sessions at weekly intervals. At the end of this time, the majority are largely symptomless. They can get into their cars. put on and tie their shoes, ride a bicycle, play a game of golf or bowl and, in fact behave like a normal human being. Not all cases are successful and these can be sent to the orthopaedic surgeon for hip replacement, but the treatment is more than often successful and most patients are very pleased with the result. Even the failures appreciate the attention they have received.

Conclusion

It will be observed that the results are largely satisfactory considering that 90% of cases so treated get some relief and only 10% are failures.

It is a satisfactory procedure and with further experience could become a very useful adjunct to surgery if it does not replace it.

In any case it is well worth a trial before any patient is referred to the surgeon.

A. Hands

Other Points I Have Found Useful for Intra-Neural Therapy

I. Treatment for resistant pain in middle finger. It sometimes occurs that injection of the posterior interosseous ganglion fails to relieve pain in the middle finger. In this case, there are two points on which one can fall back namely

(1.) posterior supraclavicular nerve over the supra spinatus bursa:

(2.) lateral antebrachial cutaneous nerve at the elbow.

2. Treatment for resistant pain in the little finger. This usually responds to injection of the dorsal branch of the ulnar. This is found just dorsal to the pisiform bone and is often noted to he tender.

B. Shoulder

1. Medial supraclavicular nerve over the shoulder joint controls pain down front of shoulder to the lateral side of arm. Usually painful as patient stretches his hand out forward to take something in front of him.

2. Points around the scapula. Tender spots are often found around and under the scapula and are probably due to nerve damage in the periscapular area. Although these can be treated by injections, they respond much better to the treatment by laser beam or acupuncture needles. They can he found at all the three corners of the scapula.

C. Hip

1 . Lower nervous branches from nerve to quadratus femoris.

There may he two, or even three of these, and they are situated along the posterior border of the femur.

2. Descending branch of the ilio-hypogastric nerve. This is found halfway between the upper border of the trocanter and the tip of the iliac crest.

D. Knee

1. The lateral cutaneous nerve of the calf (sural nerve). This is found superficial to the lateral ligament of the knee. I have found it particularly useful in overweight patients.

2. Medial and lateral eyes. At times and, especially in the very chronic case, some knees still fail to respond and I have used acupuncture points developed by them as the "medial and lateral eyes" which are on either side of the ligamentum patellae. My idea is to catch the tender nerves below the tibial plateau and then inject into the region of the cruciate ligaments. Flex the knee and then mark the spots on one or either sides of the ligament, according to which is tender. Then, with the knee flexed and the needle introduced pointing distally, advance until pain is felt. Inject 1 cc of the mixture and then withdraw the needle and introduce it into the centre of the joint, either medially in the case of the lateral eye or, laterally in the case of the medial eye. These usually solve the problem of pain in the joint during any long distance walking.

The Control of Pain in Arthritis of the Knee
by
Paul Notrik

(Pseudonym used by Dr. Paul K Pybus to avoid South African medical society accusations of "advertising" whenever a physician writes for lay people.)

Foreward

Roger Wyburn-Mason was a man of great foresight and understanding of medicine, but was born 100 years before his time. In the days when I was a House Physician I had the honour of working with him at Hounslow Hospital in 1951, and during this time I became more and more impressed with his understanding and knowledge. Many of my colleagues considered his statements way out and absurd, but I was always impressed by his ways, and he repeatedly proved himself correct.

One year before his death, he wrote an article on the manner of inflammation and gave me a copy. That treatise really says all that he fought for during his lifetime, and it embodies the basis of my beliefs. His work now makes my brain tick and on it my researches are based. I am commencing this small booklet with that unpublished writing, included as a kind of preface, with the kind permission of his widow, Joan Wyburn-Mason.

This work must not be forgotten and buried with him, and it is presented here through the enthusiasm and help of Perry A. Chapdelaine, Executive Director-Secre-tary of The Roger Wyburn-Mason and Jack M. Blount Foundation for the Eradication of Rheumatoid Disease (The Arthritis Trust of America/The Rheumatoid Disease Foundation), who has agreed to publication and to whom proceeds (donations) from its sale will be given.

The Neurogenic Nature of Inf lammation and the Existence of Trophic Ner ves in Mammals and Man

by

ROGER WYBURN-MASON

late of

National Hospital for Nervous Diseases, Queen Square, London.

Yale University Medical School, New Haven, Conn. U.S.A.

Mayo Clinic, Rochester, Minn, U.S.A. Royal Marsden Hospital, London.

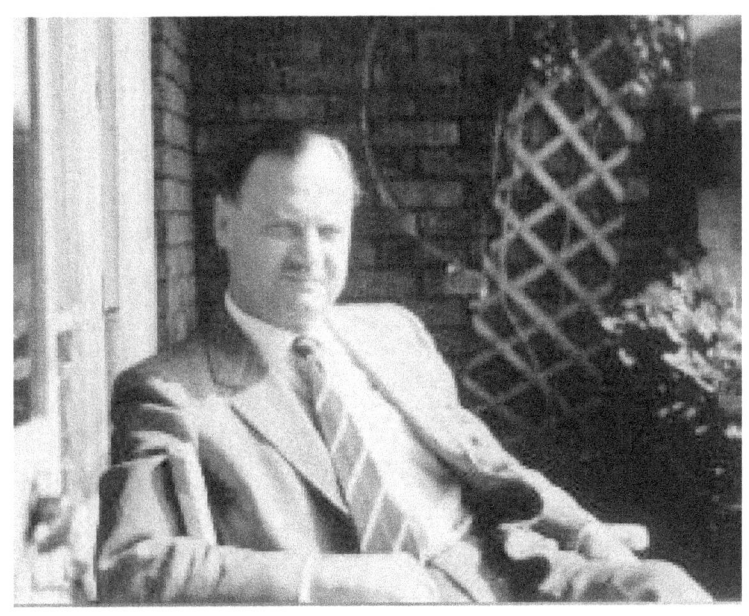

The late Professor Roger Wyburn-Mason

Type of joint	Joint pain Numbers	Numbers of Failures	Months of Relief	Average relief in (months)
Hips	37	3	385	10.4
Knees	124	7	1421	11.45
Ankles	44	5	491	11.15
Shoulders	44	1	716	16.27
Elbows	19	0	339	7.3
Hands	56	7	549	9.6
Sciatica	49	1	496	10.12
Neck	20	2	283	14.2
Totals	393	25	4740	11.31

This is a survey of one third of Dr. Pybus' patients, (A-G), treated by this method over the past 4 years. Only those patients who have been regularly followed up are included. There are many other patients whose results we do not have, as the patients have been lost to follow-up.

SUMMARY

Though accepted by early neurologists, the existence of trophic nerves has remained in doubt. Moreover, the exact nature of inflammation is not fully understood. This paper shows that trophic nerves certainly exist in the sensory nerve roots and that antidromic or reverse activity in them is responsible for inflammation and recovery from injury.

INTRODUCTION

For many years in the latter half of the last century [1800s] and the beginning of this [1900s], the idea of the existence of trophic nerves serving a protective role in the tissues was accepted, but gradually lost favour, as their minute diameters led to difficulties in demonstrating their existence. For this reason necrotic gangrenous lesions appearing in sensory denervated tissues have been attributed to neglect of unfelt injuries. Furthermore, histamine and prostaglandins are now well recognised to be liberated in areas of inflammation in animals. Most non-steroidal anti-inflammatory drugs consist of either antihistamines or substances with antiprostaglandin properties, but do not completely abolish inflammation. In order to understand the reasons for this, it is necessary to consider the following observations about the nature of inflammation.

Clinico-anatomical considerations. Experimental methods and observations.

1. Deep or slow pain is conducted by the unmyelinated C fibres of the mixed peripheral nerves having their nerve cells in the posterior nerve root ganglia. They originate in the skin and other tissues as well as the internal organs. When irritated anywhere in their length, they can transmit impulses in both forward and reverse directions. Prodromic impulses produce the sensation of slow pain by conduction of impulses along the branch axons of the posterior root ganglia cells into the cord and thence to the brain. Antidromic impulses pass to the blood vessels and other structures in the region of the peripheral origin of these nerve fibres, causing liberation of the peptide SP (a neurohormone) and leading to an increase in the blood supply, heat and oedema in these situations[5, 6, 14] being the changes of inflammation. Liberation occurs when the distal end of a freshly cut sensory nerve is stimulated in both man and animals. My late chief, Sir Thomas Lewis, in his classical monograph showed that a mild noxious stimulus to intact skin resulted in the "triple response". This consists of a local area of capillary vasodilation surrounded by one where fluid contents of the blood have leaked out through the increasingly permeable capillary walls and this again by an area of local anteriolar vasodilation or "flare". These are the fundamental changes of inflammation in miniature. The ease with which this response is induced varies with the subject's emotional state and the presence or not of neurological or mental disease (tache cerebrale), itself indicating the importance of centrifugal (antidromic or reverse) nervous impulses in the modification of the "triple response". Lewis showed that experimental section of the posterior nerve root supply to the affected area and its subsequent degeneration modified the "triple response" by abolishing the "flare" and it can be assumed that the same abolition will occur in the full-blown inflammatory response to a stimulus by suppression of "antidromic" posterior nerve root impulses.

2. The writer extended these findings by recalling that in a limb affected by causalgia, a condition resulting from damage to the sensory fibres in the median or sciatic nerves, a mild stimulus, which produces little or no observable reaction in the normal skin of the patient other than the triple response, may induce a severe and grossly excessive inflammatory reaction in the painful parts affected by the causalgia[2, 4, 9, 18].

Furthermore, the inflammatory change so produced by a mild noxious stimulus, which in normal skin shows no obvious change or a minimal triple response and rapidly returns to normal, persists in the causalgic region and even progresses to cellulitis without any attempt at healing. Again, water which is only warm and in no way painful in normal areas of skin may cause excessive inflammation and vesiculation in the painful areas, while mustard plaster applied to the affected skin blisters it more readily than in normal areas[4].

This is due to the excessive nervous activity and resultant extreme inflammation.

3. In contrast, in cases of complete section of the sciatic nerve in the thigh, any neurological textbook records that the anaesthetic areas in the foot are liable to develop painless so-called trophic sores (really atrophic) or perforating ulcers, that is, areas of gangrene (NOT inflammation) of the skin and underlying tissues, which show no attempt at healing or regeneration.

The same applies to the anaesthetic areas of the hand in cases of syringomyelia, of the feet in tabes dorsalis and the peripheries of the limbs in leprosy. Common to all lesions is destruction of the sensory nerve fibres to the affected areas. These "trophic" lesions have been wrongly attributed to neglected injury in the anaesthetic areas resulting in inflammation. Such an explanation is untenable, since, if this were correct, the trophic lesions should consist of inflammation, whereas they are areas of necrosis and really atrophy. The writer[17] showed that if a drop of mustard oil was applied to the normal skin on any of the above conditions, it produced typical transient painful inflammation, but if applied to the anaesthetic areas in the region of the trophic necrotic sores, it did not cause pain, a triple response or inflammation, but a further area of painless gangrene with no attempt at healing. The same is true of experimental sciatic nerve section in dogs[12].

4. The lens of the eye, which is the only living organ in the body which has no nerve supply, is never subject to inflammation after injury.

5. The writer[17] showed that malignant tumours have no motor or sensory nerve supply (other than those of the invaded tissue). Trauma or the application of drugs which in normal tissues

cause inflammation, such as nitrogen mustard, when applied to malignant tissue do not induce pain or inflammation, but necrosis; hence the use of such drugs in the treatment of malignancies.

6. Local anaesthetics, such as cocaine, procaine and related substances, which depress activity in peripheral nerve fibres, have been shown to be anti-inflammatory and lessen pain when applied to cases of conjunctivitis and rheumatoid arthritis. In this connection the writer had under his care two identical male twins, aged 25 years, who both developed rheumatoid arthritis at the same time and of the same severity, becoming increasingly worse in spite of identical standard treatment with the same anti-inflammatory drugs. One brother suddenly began to make dramatic improvement in his condition with disappearance of all clinical evidence of active inflammation for no obvious reason. However, the sedimentation rate remained high and the pre-existing anaemia persisted. After persistent close questioning he admitted that he had started sniffing cocaine and was now an addict. His twin's condition continued to deteriorate. This indicates that suppression of nervous impulses by local anaesthetics inhibits the inflammatory process.

CONCLUSIONS

These collected findings show that the *inflammatory response* to injury, drugs or a local infection and the *healing process* depend on an intact efferent posterior nerve root supply and is primarily reflexly neurogenically produced with the liberation of a neurohormone (SP) at the peripheral nerve endings. Liberation of prostaglandins and histamine is only of secondary importance. Inflammation does not occur in response to injury in a completely nerveless area or organ, but only gangrene and a failure to heal. On the contrary, in painful areas the inflammatory response to injury is excessive. These findings accord with the role played by intact posterior nerve root fibres in the regeneration of the distal ends of severed limbs in amphibia. Section of a single sensory nerve root, for example the trigeminal or spinal nerve, does not cause complete denervation of the corresponding tissue, since there is overlapping from neighbouring sensory nerve roots. Hence, the incompletely denervated areas are not so liable to necrosis in response to trauma as they would be if the anaesthesia was complete. Necrotic areas do occur in the trigeminal distribution in some cases of trigeminal root section. Such observations prove the existence of the once generally recognized, but now much doubted, trophic nerves.

The ideal anti-inflammatory drug would be one with an anaesthetic effect on unmyelinated C fibres (trophic nerves) or which antagonizes SP, but would not be habit forming and have side effects. Pharmaceutical firms would be wiser to spend their efforts in some direction other than producing even more anti-prostaglandins, but in any case the reason for the inflammation in rheumatoid arthritis should be first removed, but that is a separate subject[15.16].

Roger Wyburn-Mason

CHAPTER 1 **Historical**

The late Professor Roger Wyburn-Mason, the co-nominee of our foundation [Arthritis Trust of America/The Rheumatoid Disease Foundtion, AKA's for The Roger Wyburn-Mason & Jack M. Blount Foundation for the Eradication of Rheumatoid Disease], was a man of exceptional clinical acumen and observation. Way back in 1951, when I had the honour to be his House Physician, he taught me the principle that nervous activity was the prime cause of inflammation. He correctly told me that the inflammation was caused by anti-dromic impulses travelling along the damaged unmyelinated nerve fibres to the periphery in the joint, quoting Sir Thomas Lewis as his reference. Furthermore, he was able to demonstrate time and again that certain nerves were exquisitely tender to the touch. He gave these nerve fibres, probably unfortu-nately, the name "*trophic nerves*". This was received with disbelief, as there existed at the time ulcers known as "*trophic ulcers*", which had been shown conclusively to possess no nerves, as they were painless. Their proper name should have been "*atrophic ulcers*", as they had no trophic nerves in them. This, however, was not fully recognised at the time.

For the purpose of this manual, I will stick to the term "*trophic nerve*", but the reader must understand that these nerves are identical with the C-type dorsal root fibre or Type IV of the numerical classification as sometimes used. Further reference will be made to them in later chapters.

During my stay in Hounslow Hospital, I learnt from Dr. Wyburn-Mason that blocking these nervous impulses from their inflamed trophic nerves produced truly remarkable effects. I was taught and shown how to treat successfully, at the time, substantially untreatable conditions like sciatica, trigeminal neuralgia, migraine, intermittent claudication, facial palsy and many forms of intractable pain by means of blocking these trophic nerves. Also at this time we started to investigate methods of suppressing nervous activity to various joints in the treatment of arthritis, the most notable, to my mind, being the complete relief of pain and stiffness of the arthritic hand.

In those days, cortisone had not been fully developed and for the purpose of blocking these nerves, dehydrated alcohol was used. This procedure was extremely painful but remarkably effective in all cases.

At the end of my sojourn at Hounslow, both Wyburn-Mason and myself went our separate ways, Wyburn-Mason to greater research in an attempt to expound his ideas to an unbelieving profession, whilst I proceeded into the realms of general surgery, which took me to many corners of the globe. Although I have always been engaged in seeing and treating surgical patients, I never really forgot the teaching of Wyburn-Mason, and the remarkable results that he could produce.

It was not until 1978, when advancing presbyopia had whispered to me to abandon surgery and enter general practice, that I made my remarkable discovery, which I shall describe in some detail.

I had taken on the post of District Surgeon and this position included the duties of caring for the elderly indigent patients of my area. Many of these people suffered terribly with osteoarthritis of the knees, and each of my colleagues from whom I sought advice proposed a different anti-inflammatory drug, each of which I tried in turn. I was bombarded by medical reps, each promoting his own particular product with great zeal and enthusiasm. Each of the non steroidal anti-inflammatory drugs I tried in turn proved the same dismal failure, as not only was the pain not substantially relieved, but many developed the side effects of gastric upsets and in some cases gastric ulceration. I had had one serious haematemis from the use of one of these drugs.

Then one summer's day I had a visit from a medical representative from Sherag who was conducting a promotion of the depot steroid of B-methazone known as Celestone Soluspan. He suggested that I should inject this substance into the knee joint of patients, telling me that I could relieve their pain for several months at a time. He gave me details and statistics to prove his point and left me the usual supply of samples.

I was really not very impressed, as I knew that this procedure was often done but had to be performed under strict, aseptic conditions and not in the doctor's surgery, for the penalty for infection would be high.

Two days later, a 68-year-old crippled, overweight lady came to my surgery, hobbling in on two sticks and complaining of severe pain in her right knee, from which she had suffered for the last 10 years. The knee was swollen and very painful and kept her awake at night. She was quite unable to get around to any extent, and had to have a stick for every step she took. Examination showed her to have a marked degree of knock-knee and there was an effusion present.

She had come asking for her repeat supply of pills for sleeping, and for hyper-tension, from which she also suffered, and anti-inflammatory drugs. I proceeded to write out her prescription, and as I was doing this she said to me, "You know, Doctor, I'm sure if you put something in just here" (pointing to the medial side of the knee below the medial tibial condyle), "I am sure you would help me a great deal." "All right," I said, "show me and get up on the couch."

After great deal of puffing and blowing and wincing at the pain, this tired, obese old lady managed to lie down on the couch in the supine position and point to the inner side of the knee, saying "There, Doctor."

It was only then that I remembered the visit of my medical-rep friend and his sample of Celestone Soluspan. I had previously injected this material into tender points around the shoulder and wondered if I could do it in this condition. I knew that the injection, if used as presented by the makers, was very painful, so I thought it would be kinder to dilute it, as this spot was very tender indeed. I therefore used 2% lignocaine which I discovered in another corner of the surgery, and drew up 5 ml. of this. I then raised a bleb of anaesthetic over the tender spot and then to the remainder of the lignocaine added 1 ml. of the Celestone Soluspan. I then introduced the solution into the spot and advanced the needle further into the skin. The old lady winced a little, but made no fuss, saying it was just a little painful.

When I had completed the injection I felt the joint and tried to bend it. To my surprise a miracle had occurred. Instead of the patient experiencing severe pain and resistance to movement as had occurred previously, the knee flexed with the greatest of ease to full flexion, and her expression changed from one of painful anticipation to one of satisfied pleasure. It was difficult to tell who was the most surprised, the patient or myself. Neither of us could really believe that such a God-sent miracle had occurred. Although I did not see my face, I felt tears come into my eyes as I saw the ecstacy in her face. I flexed the knee again and there was still no pain. I could not believe it. I wondered if I had inadvertently given the mixture intravenously and it had had some peculiar effect that I did not understand, but the pulse and heart beat were normal. I asked her to stand up. This she did, and to our surprise there was still no pain. She then asked for her sticks, which I gave her. She took one step and then two, and said: "I don't want these sticks anymore, I am better now"; and with that, walked to the other end of the room and back with a smile of satisfaction on her face.

I then asked her to sit down and tested her skin sensitivity which was still intact as the skin sensitivity is at first not affected (see later). I then told her to go home and come back the next day.

The next day she returned, still wearing a big smile, saying she still had no pain, only a small bruise. Her knee still showed full painless flexion and she was walking well.

Four days later an elderly Indian lady came to see me with a similar story of osteoarthritis of the right knee. She also used a stick and could hardly get up the two steps into the surgery. She had suffered for 6 years and the usual treatment had proved ineffective. This time I palpated her saphenous nerve below the tibial condyle and found it to be exquisitely tender. I used another ampoule of my friend's Celestone Soluspan sample in the identical way.

The result was the same. The relief was immediate, the flexion and the extension full, and she was able to go down the steps without pain.

Both these patients 5 years later are able to walk around freely, without pain, and are not taking analgesics or antiarthritic drugs of any sort.

Ten days later it was a Sunday. My right knee, which was badly damaged in a motor-car accident 29 years ago, subsequently required a patellectomy, and I was told at the time that I had early osteoarthritis. On this Sunday, I was afflicted by severe pain in that knee. I had distinct tenderness along the saphenous nerve and the joint felt extremely stiff. This impeded my normal progress and I had to use a stick to get up some steps from my house. I managed to get into my car and drive over to the surgery and sat in my consulting room. I then marked the area of tenderness over the saphenous nerve, screwed up my courage, and injected myself, raising a bleb of local anaesthetic. I then added the third of my friend's samples to the local and advanced the needle gingerly towards where I thought the saphenous nerve lay.

At first I felt nothing, then suddenly there was a sharp jab of pain. I injected the mixture and the pain immediately became momentarily worse. I can only describe the feeling that then followed as one of ecstatic relief. This severe pain seemed to melt away and the whole area which was previously so painful became numb. It was a fantastic feeling and one I shall never forget. I injected the whole 5 ml., put down the syringe, applied a dressing and stood up. There was no pain. I felt the knee. It was absolutely pain-free and I could no longer feel the crepitation. I started to walk. It was easy and painless. I could not believe it even though I had two other patients who had had the same experience. I put the instruments away, closed the surgery door, got back into the car and drove home. It was only at this stage that I noticed the inner portion of my leg becoming insensitive to pinprick, which formerly it was not. I did not really know what would happen next, but I walked around normally for the next 5 hours, still without pain as the knee was still anaesthetized.

At the end of this period I suddenly realised that I could now feel normal sensation and pricked myself with a pin to confirm this. The anaesthetic had worn off but my arthritis pain had gone! There was just a small bruise where I had put the injection but this did not hurt. I went and thanked God for sending me this comfort, and from that moment I was inspired and determined to tell the whole world about this. I have tried to do this ever since, and that is the reason for this booklet.

Since that time I have treated over 2,000 knees by this method. They have all responded in the same way. Some recur in a few days, others in weeks or months or years, but it matters not. It is merely necessary to repeat the injection and the same result occurs.

I have done no double-blind experiments as I fail to see what advantage there could be in such a trial. It is not a method to advertise the efficacy of any particular drug, but to promote a technique. It is suggested by some of my colleagues and others that I should inject water as a placebo. Has this been done before? I can find no reference to it and I doubt that it would work. Such an action, in my estimation, is unjustified and unethical. Our calling is to cure patients and not to experiment in this fashion. I leave this idea to others.

CHAPTER 2

The Present Position

Osteoarthritis, osteoarthrosis or degenerative joint disease is a painful, degenerative condition affecting mainly the larger weight-bearing joints and resulting in erosion of the cartilage (osteoarthrosis) and inflammation of the synovia (osteoarthritis).

It usually follows one large traumatic incident or a series of minor traumata over a longer period. In a typical case the patient complains of a stiff joint in the morning on waking, and it may also be painful. During the day, the stiffness often passes off so that by mid-morning the joint may approach normality. Later in the day the joint becomes more painful and by the evening it is most severe. Movements of the joint are often accompanied by crepitus (creaking), of which the patient may also complain. The pain is relieved by rest and warm and dry climatic conditions as well as by pressure bandaging, and is exacerbated by exercise, cold and wet conditions and injury.

Examination shows the affected joint to be swollen. Passive movement of the joint reveals that the muscles are tight and in spasm and the joint can be moved only with difficulty against resistance which elicits pain and crepitus. Palpation around the joint shows spots of intense tenderness, the significance of which will be discussed later.

The treatment at present, apart from major surgical intervention, is mainly palliative. The patient is instructed to lose weight, take less exercise, avoid trauma and damp, take pain-killers and anti-inflammatory drugs and learn to live with his disease. The effectiveness of intra-articular cortisone or radioactive isotopes is not only limited but use is not without risk and is only effective in some cases.

Close examination of the tender spots found around the joint shows a close correlation with the position of superficial cutaneous sensory nerves at places where they are susceptible to trauma. They also have marked correlation to better-known acupuncture points. In the case of the knee, the saphenous nerve at the lower attachment to the medial longitudinal ligament is uniformly exquisitely tender. Further detailed palpation along the course of the nerve would sense greater stress as the knee is forcibly abducted and externally rotated (Fig 2.1), the action which is the usual method of trauma. These

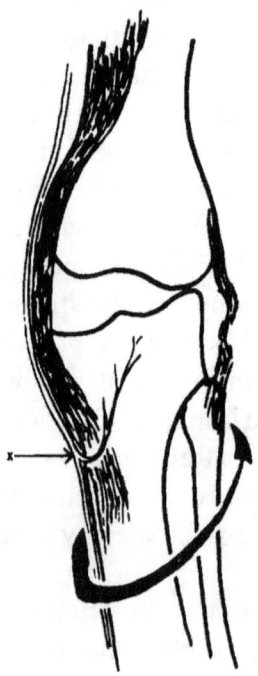

Figure 2.1

Mode of nerve injury. Diagram shows the relationship of the saphenous nerve to the lower attachment of the medial longitudinal ligament of the knee. The point of rupture and the proximity of the saphenous nerve and its infrapatellar branch are shown at point X. The direction of the strain is shown by the large arrow.

points are where the nerve is at the apex of its curve on the joint level, where its infrapatellar branch arises and at its entrance to the subsartorial canal.

In addition there are other nerves in the area that are tender, namely the external femoral cutaneous nerve as it pierces the deep fascia, the intermediate femoral cutaneous nerve on the outer side of the patella, the infrapatellar branch of the saphenous nerve below the tibial plateau. All these points are clearly shown in Fig 2.2 and every case examined will show at least one of them to be tender, and often more than one.

Each of these tender spots is marked with a skin pencil. A bleb of local anaesthetic is raised at the marked spots (Fig 2.3); a Dermo jet vaccinator (Fig 2.4) can be used for the purpose, as the injection is then painless. Through each anaesthetized bleb, the injection needle is introduced towards the suspected location of the nerve, and the patient's face is watched at the same time. At some stage the patient's facial expression changes and the doctor will see before he needs to be told when his needle is in the correct place. At this very instant the injection of a mixture of 4.5 ml. 1% local anaesthetic and 0.5 ml. depot steroid is introduced.

At this stage, the patient, although experiencing severe pain, at the same time feels this very pain melt away and the whole knee takes on a numb feeling. Watching the patient's face show successive expressions of anticipation, expectation, configuration and realization that the pain has gone is the chief joy for the doctor who performs this procedure. An attempt is now made to flex the knee, and one that was previously stiff and painful is now found to be loose and painless.

It is well to have small dressings available, as these injection sites often show marked capillary oozings and each point should be covered with a dressing which remains in situ until this bleeding has stopped. The increased oozing is probably due to the local production of prostaglandins.

The patient is now able to get up and is told to walk around the surgery. The improvement is immediately apparent to the patient, who no longer has any pain, and to the doctor who observes the improved walking.

It must be explained that the numb feeling is only temporary and that in about five hours the normal sensitivity returns, with the injection site being tender due to bruising, but that the arthritic pain will no longer he present. The patient is also warned not to do rash things in his new-found freedom from pain during these five hours, but to proceed with his normal activities. It must he remembered that there is no sensitivity in the joint at this time, as it is temporarily in a "Charcot state," and so unnecessary trauma must be avoided.

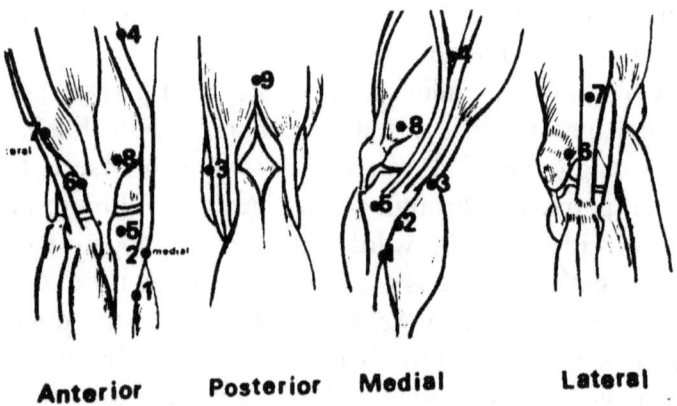

Anterior   Posterior   Medial   Lateral

Figure 2.2
Sites for intraneural injections for the arthritic knee.

1. *Saphenous nerve at the lower attachment of the medial longitudinal ligament.*
2. *Saphenous nerve at the origin of the infrapatellar branch.*
3. *Saphenous nerve at the knee-joint level.*
4. *Saphenous nerve as it enters the subsartorial canal.*
5. *Infrapatellar branch of the saphenous nerve.*
6. *Intermediate femoral cutaneous nerve.*
7. *External femoral cutaneous nerve.*
8. *Medial femoral cutaneous nerve.*
9. *Posterior femoral cutaneous nerve.*

The next week the patient returns to the surgery and the knee is examined again and any further tender spots are sought and, if found, similarly treated. He is seen weekly until the knee is painless. Two or three visits are usually sufficient. The treatment can be repeated as often as required.

It will be noticed during this time that not only is the knee getting less painful, less stiff and exhibiting less crepitus, but the patient is walking better, sleeps better and has little to no pain. His friends are truly amazed, as they have watched him abandon his sticks, take brisker walks and even resume some of his sporting activities. No longer do they have to listen to his moans and groans about his arthritis, but instead to his recovery story. A new life has been opened up for him.

Over the past 6 years I have treated over 2,000 knees with almost universal success. My practice grows daily but is not

unmanageable as the patient is rapidly cured, and then only seen once a year or less frequently than this.

Initial Bleb

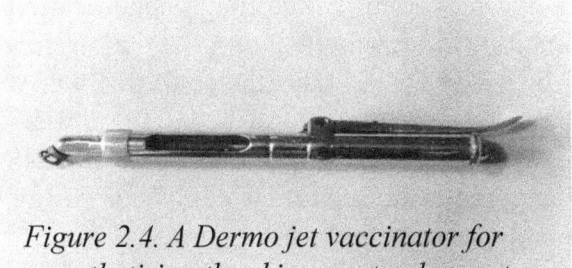

Figure 2.4. A Dermo jet vaccinator for anesthetizing the skin over tender spots.

CHAPTER 3

Theory and Explanation

At this stage in my research it was necessary to produce some form of theory to support my findings scientifically, and my first assignment was to read up on the subject as thoroughly as possible and to weave together the various facts and observations that I could find in the literature.

NUTRITION OF ARTICULAR CARTILAGE

There are no blood vessels in articular cartilage. Rather, nutrient fluids reach the cartilage cells by two main routes, namely, diffusion from the vascularisal bone marrow at the cartilaginous base, and circulation of the synovial fluid at the articular surface of the cartilage. McCutchen[8] described the cartilage as acting like a sponge which is alternately squeezed free of synovial fluid during weight bearing and then soaks it up on relaxation. Impairment of nutrition can lead to cartilage destruction, as can be shown by the experiments of compression fixation shown below.

EXPERIMENTAL PRODUCTION OF OSTEOARTHRITIS

In the early part of the 1960's several investigators quite independently explored the effect of continuous compression exerted on the joint cartilage.

Robert Salter and Paul Field[10] working in Toronto, Antoni Trias[13] in Oxford, and Crelin and Southwick[3] in Cambridge, Mass. were all performing experiments on the knee joints of either monkeys or rabbits. Their experiments were essentially similar in the principle of using a Charnley's clamp to be applied across one knee joint of a large number of animals for a number of days (Fig 3.1). After the application of the clamp, the animals were allowed to recover from the anaesthetic, and thereafter one was sacrificed every day and the joint fixed in formalin and examined microscopically. The opposite knee was used as the control.

All these investigations obtained essentially similar results. An osteoarthritic-type lesion, including prominent cartilage degeneration was produced in the joint following as few as 3 days continuous fixation-compression, and by the end of 14 days the condition was well established. After 6 weeks the joint degeneration was in its final stages, the cartilaginous joint surface being worn away with eburnation of the underlying bony layers.

It was also shown by two other workers, Calandruccio and Gilmer[1] that this experimental fixation-compression is released, the condition is reversible and the cartilage shows signs of regeneration. These workers postulated that constant fixation and compression of the joint surfaces acts by impairing nutrition of the cartilage cells.

Corresponding observations have been made in man. Specifically, orthopaedic surgeons have often noted that any continual sustained pressure applied to joints during the course of fracture treatment results in osteoarthritis developing in these joints. A good example is the "well leg" traction treatment for intertrochanteric fracture of the neck of the femur. This results in osteoar- thritis developing in the knee of the unfractured side due to the pressure on that knee exerted by the apparatus. *(Fig 3.2)*

JOINT FIXATION AND COMPRESSION IN ARTHRITIS

It is obvious from clinical observations of patients with osteoarthritis that joint pain and stiffness leads to at least partial joint fixation. Chronic spasm in the musculature surrounding the affected joint also contributes to continuing but intermittent compression. This is exacerbated by frequent obesity of the patient, this also being a well known predisposing cause. It is probable, there- fore, that chronic partial joint fixation and compression lead secondarily to degeneration of the cartilage. By this line of reasoning, relief of the pain and spasm might be expected to arrest or perhaps even reverse degeneration.

CHAPTER 4

Origin of pain and spasm through nervous disturbances

The normal nervous unit or neuron consists of a nerve cell with a nucleus with large granular cytoplasm. From this nerve cell projects a large number of dendrites which intertwine with dendrites and axons of other nerve cells. One of the projections is larger and longer than the others and is known as the axon. The cytoplasm is clearer at its origin, and is long, straight and unbranching, tracking either to the effector organ, as in the case of a motor branch, or with the receptor organ in the case of a sensory nerve.

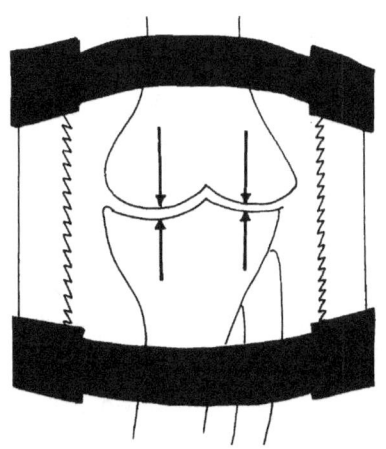

Fig 3.1:Charnley's Clamp

Normally the motor-nerve impulse is initiated in the cell and transmitted to the effector organ in the muscle, causing it to contract. The sensory impulse originates in the receptor organ at the periphery, as in the skin or synovium, and a nerve impulse is likewise created and travels to the cell. The impulse normally only travels in one direction, namely peripherally in the case of motor impulses, or centrally as in the case of the sensory ones.

THE NORMAL SPINAL REFLEX

All sensory impulses arise from a receptor organ, the most prominent of which are the plain nerve receptor organs, found in the skin and synovium amongst other places. These, when stimulated, initiate an impulse which travels centrally to the spinal cord and, where after being modified by the cell in the spinal cord, eventually sets off an impulse in the appropriate motor-nerve cell. This impulse travels peripherally to the muscle, which contracts to remove the threatened area from the painful stimulus. This is a very simplified explanation of what occurs. Only by stimulating either the motor-nerve cell or the receptor organ is it possible to produce a stimulus in a normal nerve. Normal stimulation of an intact, undamaged nerve will not produce any impulse.

The normal impulse is not to be regarded as a message travelling down a telephone wire as is often suggested. The impulse is an active process involving intricate electrical and chemical changes in the nerve, and should be likened to lighting a trail of gunpowder, ignited at one end, and travelling by the active process of burning to the other. After the impulse has been conducted, the axon, after a latent period of inactivity, is repaired and another trail is laid for the next impulse. This all occurs in a fraction of a second. Thus, normally the impulse travels rapidly in one direction only, namely a central direction in the sensory nerves and a peripheral direction in the motor nerves.

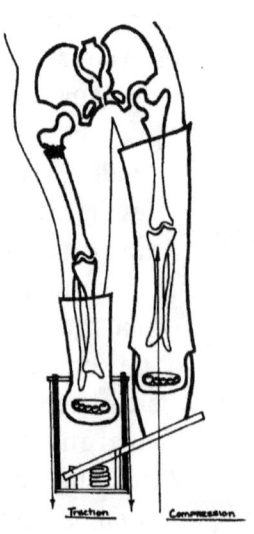

Figure 3.2.

The "well leg" traction. Osteoarthritis develops in the knee of the unfractured side due to the pressure on that knee exerted by the apparatus.

If a normal C-type sensory nerve (trophic nerve) is damaged, however, this area of damage becomes negative due to the disturbance in its sheath, and also becomes a local generator of electrical impulses, and in this situation the impulse will travel not only in the normal or prodromic direction, but also in the opposite peripheral or antidromic direction.

Thus, using the same analogy of the gunpowder trail, if the impulse starts in the centre of the trail, it will burn in both directions at the same time; and what is more, these impulses are given off at frequent intervals so that there is a constant barrage of impulses in both directions.

The prodromic impulses are conducted to the spinal cord where they communicate with the motor neurons, likewise giving off numerous impulses to cause spasm of the musculature (Fig 4.1). This spasm causes the joint surfaces to be compressed together and cause damage to the underlying cartilage as described in the previous chapter. This is known as osteoarthrosis. The barrage of antidromic impulses travel peripherally, and it was shown many years ago by Sir Thomas Lewis[7] that these antidromic impulses produce distal inflammation, this being known as osteoarthritis.

It is a constant argument as to whether the condition should be known as osteoarthritis or osteoarthrosis, some preferring one term and some the other, but it will be seen now that both are probably correct.

CHAPTER 5

Electrical Disturbances in Nerves

It has been proven over the years that definite electrical currents flow along nerves during the passage of an impulse. Microsurgery has been performed on the nerve fibres of the squid. These nerves are very large having semi-solid interiors and an outer membrane. It has been shown conclusively that the interior part of the axon is negatively charged whilst the outer membrane is positively charged. If a micro-electrode is introduced into the tube and the other electrode is placed on the surface, and both connected to a galvanometer, there is a definite flow of current from the negatively charged interior to the positively charged exterior (Fig 5.1).

Normally the membrane is impervious to electrons, so no current flows. If, however, there is a temporary increased permeability in the sheath, as occurs with a normal impulse, then there is a flow of current out of the negative axon to the positive exterior (Fig 5.2). This is a normal method of the propagation of a nervous impulse.

When the nerve fibre is damaged, an electrical disturbance occurs as electrons leak through the membrane and cause a negatively charged area around the damage, and this in itself acts as a generator of electrical stimuli to travel along the positively charged sheath in both antidromic and prodromic directions (Fig 5.3).

These now-ectopic electrons will be responsible for the barrage of impulses described earlier. In order that the ectopic impulse should cease, it is necessary either that these negatively charged electrons should be removed or that the leak from the sheath should be stopped. and this can be done in one of two ways to be described later.

To summarize, therefore, I would propose that the nerve is primarily damaged and from this area of damage an electrical disturbance is created, resulting in both prodromic and antidromic impulses along the nerve. The antidromic impulses are conducted peripherally to the synovial membrane where they cause an inflammation or arthritis, whilst the prodromic impulses are conducted centrally to the spinal cord where they relay with the motor nerves to cause muscle spasm. This muscular spasm causes compression of the cartilaginous surfaces which interferes with the nutrition of the cells of the cartilage and produces death of the cells and an arthrosis.

Two methods of reversing this condition will now be described.

CHAPTER 6

Method for reversing electrical nervous disturbances

As discussed in previous chapters, there is a leak of electrons or negatively charged particles from the inside of the nerve fibre to the outside, so that the whole of the area around the damaged nerve has a negative charge.

Thus there are obviously two possible methods of reducing the negativity of this area. namely:

1.Removal of the electrons.

This is often done today by the use of acupuncture needles. These needles are fine-pointed needles, made of a metal that has a good conductivity of electricity. They can be made of gold, which is the best conductor, or silver, but to avoid expense are usually made from stainless steel.

These needles act like a miniature lightning conductor in the tissues, as they have a small receptor area in the form of a point and electrons will be attracted to this point, just as a lightning conductor attracts electrons out of the atmosphere and returns them

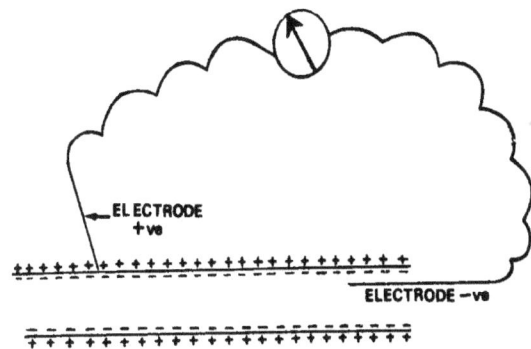

Electrical Potential for Normal Nerve

Figure 5.1

The flow of current along an axon from the negatively charged interior to the positively charged exterior.

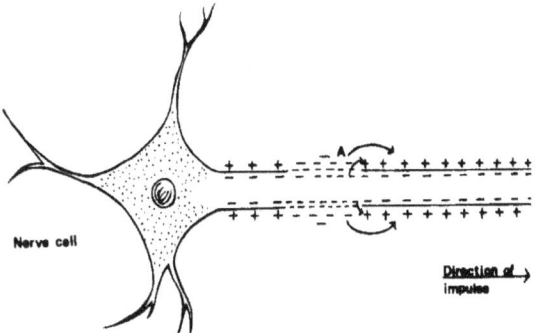

Figure 5.2

Electrical changes occurring with a normal impulse the direction for which is clearly shown.

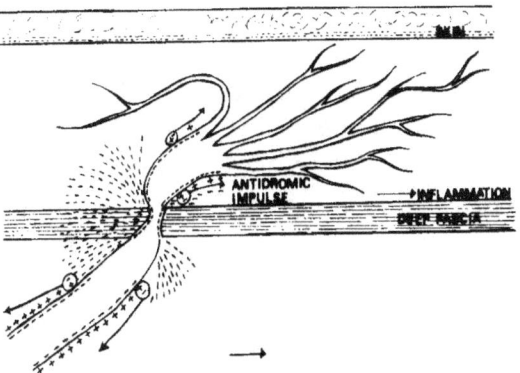

Figure 5.3

Shows damage to the nerve by constriction in tissue, and shows leak of negative electrons.

to earth. The same occurs in the human body, and such a case is shown in Fig. 6.1 a,b,c,d. Fig. 6 a will show the patient with a severe limitation of movement of the right shoulder, 6 b, after **2. Blocking and repair of the defect in the nerve membrane.**

To oppose and reverse this inflammation, it is necessary to introduce some local anaesthetic such as procaine or lignocaine. These substances act as what is known as a membrane stabilizer, that is, they prevent the passage of electrons through the membrane and so effectively stop the passage of nervous impulses. Different types of nerve fibres become anaesthetised at different rates, depending on the thick- ness of the sheath through which the local anaesthetic has to penetrate. As theC-type fibres (trophic nerves) are remarkable for their thin membrane, they are anaesthetised immediately, while the thicker A-type fibre, responsible for skin sensation, is anaesthetised only after about 10 minutes. This would explain the slow onset of loss of pinprick sensation that occurs during the treatment. Thus it will be seen that the suppression of the nervous activity at the site of the damaged nerve will immediately stop the pain, and immediately reflexly abolish the muscular spasm, which in point of fact is what is observed. Unfortunately, however, the local will last only for a few hours, after which time the position is reversed and the inflamed area still present, so that with the use of local alone the symptoms will return. The defect in the nerve membrane has been blocked only temporarily and not repaired.

The repair of this defect can only he achieved by suppressing the inflammatory reaction, and this is where the use of an anti-inflammatory agent is involved. The most powerful anti-inflammatory agents are the steroids, and I use these in preference to the anti-inflammatory drugs for two reasons:

1) They are very effective.
2) They are the only ones made in depot form.

When an injection is made in a depot form, the active substance is released very slowly from the site of injection, and the action is almost entirely local. This has a great advantage over the other routes as the active substance acts only where it is injected and nowhere else to any great extent. There can be no systemic side effects and none have been observed in my series of patients treated by this method, with numbers now running into thousands. The treatment is perfectly safe. The steroid is slowly released and acts

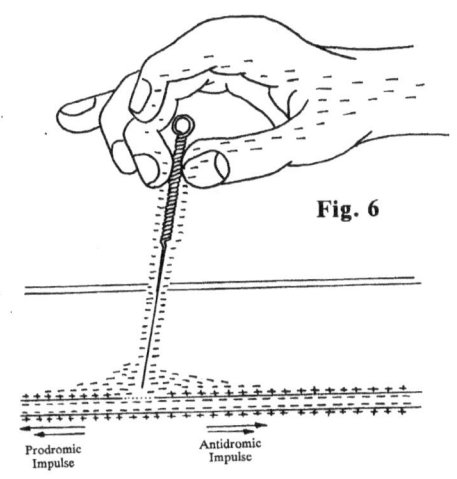

Fig. 6

Prodromic Impulse   Antidromic Impulse

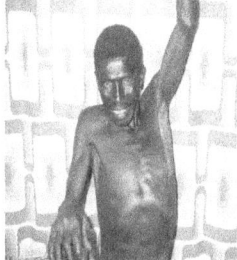

Figure 6.1a

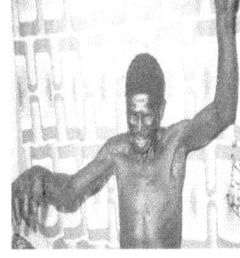

Figure 6.1c

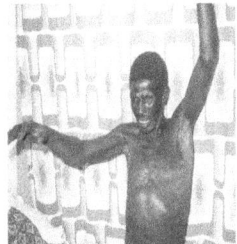

Figure 6.1b

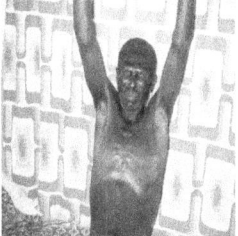

Figure 6.1d

the insertion of acupuncture needles, and 6c, when these same needles had been earthed. A progressive improvement is very obvious.

Thus, when an acupuncture needle is inserted, the electrons are immedately attracted to the point and conducted up the handle of the needle to the body of the operator to restore electrical balance (Fig 6.2). These electrons are now distributed to earth by the feet. I have found that my acupuncture results are greatly improved by the simple expediency of removing my shoes, and this may well account for the superior results obtained by the Chinese, who are usually barefoot, as opposed to those obtained by the shoe-wearing western doctor.

2. Blocking and Repair of the defect in the nerve membrane.

The defect in the nerve sheath has been caused either by trauma in the form of stretching of the nerve, as in osteoarthritis, or by invsion of [microrganisms] in the case of rheumatoid arthritis. This trauma or invasion produces a minute area of inflammation of the nerve, or neuritis.

directly on the damaged nerve to produce healing within 5 hours and then keeps it healed.

The relief lasts anywhere between 2 days and 6 years; the average period of relief is about 11 months. It matters little, however, as the injection can be easily repeated with the same beneficial effects should the pain return.

To illustrate the point better: in an earlier chapter I mentioned my own knee which was treated 6 years ago. The relief lasted 3

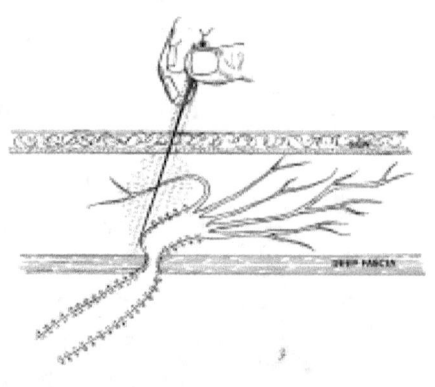

months and then I repeated the procedure, and it lasted another 3 months; I repeated it again, and the third injection lasted one year.

The final one was given 4½ years ago. I am still out of pain and get around normally. The Indian lady I also described only had the one injection, and 5½ years later is still free of pain and walks many miles a day to do her shopping. She is extremely happy.

I will not pretend that all cases are 100% successful, but the dissatisfied patients cannot be more than 15 in number, and all these considered the procedure well worth the try. At least they had found someone who was willing to do something to rid them of their agony and suffering.

It is easy to show interest if this method is tried. The method is simple if the instructions are followed carefully. Many people will be made happy, and many doctors will find great joy in their new work.

CHAPTER 7
Summary of Hypothesis on Cause of Osteoarthritis

To recapitulate what has already been said, we can now state the following: The primary lesion in the condition is one of trauma to a nonmyelinated C-type sensory nerve fibre which in this booklet we have agreed to call a trophic nerve. This trophic nerve gives off barrages of both antidromic and prodromic impulses due to the electrical changes described in Chapter 6.

The antidromic-impulse barrage is directed peripherally to the synovium of the joint to cause an increase in production of S.P. substance, which is closely related to histamine. This substance causes vasodilation, oedema, increased synovial fluid production and effusion. This produces all the properties of inflammation or osteoarthritis.

The prodromic-impulse barrage is directed centrally and, after relaying and modification in the spinal cord, is transmitted to the ventral horn cells producing a barrage of impulses conducted to the surrounding musculature and causing spasm of these muscles.

This spasm produces compression of the joint surfaces, thus preventing the proper circulation of the synovial fluid and the nutrients to the cartilage cells. These cells consequently are deprived of oxygen and are unable to rid themselves of accumulated carbon dioxide and other products of metabolism. They thus tend to die and become dissolved, with resultant thinning of the cartilage layer or osteoarthrosis.

If we accept this hypothesis, and there is much evidence in its favour, then the treatment which I have already described is obvious, namely, the suppression of the ectopic nervous impulses arising from the damaged trophic nerve.

Either these electrons can be earthed to an acupuncture needle, or the leak can be stopped by a membrane stabilizer like a local anaesthetic. If either approach is used then the symptoms will at once disappear, and this is what happens in both cases. The addition of an anti-inflammatory agent (and the best one available is a depot cortisone) will heal the breach in the membrane and restore normality.

If the breach is permanently plugged, then the causative factors will be removed and the whole process will be reversed. This is what in point of fact happens, which will now be shown by a few individual case histories taken at random from our books.

CHAPTER X

Case Histories

Mrs. H.C., aged 64, is a headmaster's wife who takes a lot of interest in the school and is continually running functions. She is also keen on gardening and walking, but had had an osteoarthritic right knee on and off for 20 years. This had been diagnosed several times by orthopaedic surgeons, and X-rays had confirmed the diagnosis. She had been treated by intra-articular injections of cortisone, as well as with many anti-inflammatories, none of which had had any great effect. She had also been given short-wave diathermy, but this had made the knee worse. The pain kept her awake at night. In her past history, she had fractured her right ankle as a girl.

On examination, the right knee was swollen and was extremely stiff with marked crepitus. She had a slight degree of tenderness over the right saphenous nerve, which was injected with 10 mgs. Lederspan* (*Editor's Note: Aristospan® is the American equivalent of Lederspan.mixed with 2% local anaesthetic.) The relief was immediate; the stiffness passed off together with the pain. Since that time 2 years ago, she has had no further trouble, apart from one slight exacerbation of the pain, but this settled spontaneously. She now does her own gardening, walks 6 kilometres with ease, and finds getting out of her car and chair very easy, and the knees are no longer stiff.

Mrs. M.T., aged 54. This slightly over-weight lady had noticed increased pain in the left knee on walking. This had been particularly severe over the past 2 months, though she had had it previously for some time. She noticed it if she wore high-heeled shoes, when the pain was very much worse. She complained that the knee was always stiff, and she could no longer sit on her haunches to do the gardening. In her past history, she had had a tennis elbow one year previously, and a frozen shoulder which lasted 6 months. She had received no treatment for the knee apart from hot baths and embrocation. At times she was unable to come down stairs in the normal manner but had to come one step at a time.

On examination, the left knee was swollen, and there was tenderness over the saphenous nerve and its infrapatellar branch. Both these spots were marked and treated with local anaesthetic and depot steroid. The next day she complained of severe pain at the site of injection due to a good deal of bruising. However, after a few days the pain went off completely and she never had any further arthritic pain.

She has attended me regularly over the past 2½ years when she has been treated for mild hypertension, and during this time has had no further trouble with her knee. Unfortunately, 32½ months after the original injection she fell over and knocked her knee again, and it became tender and painful. The saphenous nerve was noticed to be tender once more, and this was again injected; she has had no further trouble since. She walks many miles a day.

Mr. E.F.G., aged 80, was a retired farmer, who in his younger days had received many injuries to his right knee and back when involved in rugby and polo. This included a tear of his right medial cartilage, which had been removed 14 years before. He had also had a laminectomy 12 years previously, for a prolapsed intervertebral disc of L5-S1.

He now complained of severe pain and stiffness of his right knee, which forced him to lead a very sedentary life. He was unable to walk without sticks, and the pain was severe at night, disturbing his sleep. He found going up stairs nearly impossible, and was forced to use a stick for each step. He actually walked into the surgery using two sticks.

On examination, the knee was very swollen, and there was marked crepitus and severe pain on any attempt at movement. Feeling around the joint showed severe tenderness over the saphenous nerve, as described in the previous chapters. The left knee was also involved in the process, but not nearly so advanced, and he could actually stand on this leg without much pain. The right knee was treated by intra-neural injection of Celestone Soluspan and local, with the result that the stiffness and pain passed off at once, and he was immediately able to stand up and walk away, no longer using a stick at all. A week later he returned saying that the right knee was still symptom-less, but he now noticed pain in his left knee. This was likewise treated by the same method.

He remained symptomless for the next month, when he had an attack of "flu," and enforced bed rest caused the pain to return. It was again treated by the same method and he was once more able to walk around without pain.

He did not complain of his knee again until 4 months later, when I was called to see him at his home, where he had sprained his knee in a fall. He was once more severely tender over the saphenous nerve. This was again injected, and once more he was able to walk without aid, seeing me to my car which was parked in his yard.

Two months later he arrived outside my surgery, having been driven there by his wife. He had again sprained his knee, and was quite unable to get out of the car, due to the intense agony of trying to move his right leg. This forced me to see him in the automobile, and, sitting in the driver's seat, I managed to give him another intra-neural injection into his saphenous nerve. He was then completely relieved of his pain, and was able to get out of the car easily and walk into my surgery.

He remained symptomless for a further 7 months, when he had another flare-up. An X-ray taken on this occasion showed the presence of a loose body in the joint, but he refused surgical treatment and said he would prefer to be treated as he was.

After that date, he attended at roughly 6-monthly intervals for further injections into his saphenous nerve, and he died 2 years later of a cerebal thrombosis, but with a symptomless knee.

Mrs. N.V.F., aged 60, was a keen tennis player, and complained of pain and stiffness of the right knee. This had started 8 years ago when she fell on her knee playing tennis, and she was now unable to play, as she could not straighten the knee. She also had trouble with bunions on both feet; these had been operated on by an orthopaedic surgeon, but were, however, still painful, and she was certainly unable to run.

On examination she was hypertensive, blood pressure 200/100, and the right knee was extremely stiff, showing five degrees of fixed flexion, the crepitus being very marked. Both feet were extremely tender, the left being worse than the right. She was markedly tender over both saphenous nerves, and also over the central femoral cutaneous nerve of the right leg. She was quite unable to extend the knee fully. Both saphenous nerves were injected at the angle between the tibial condyle and the tibial shaft. These injections were slightly painful but at the end of the injections, both knees took on a numb sensation. She was seen again one week later, when she had no pain at all, and the right knee could now be fully extended. Crepitus was also considerably less, and her blood pressure had fallen to 140/90.

She was seen again one week later, and the crepitus was hardly discernable.

She was not seen again until exactly one year later. She said that she had been well until 2 months previously when she had had slight pain in the right knee, and this had temporarily removed her from the tennis court! During this time she had only taken one Indocid, and no pain-killers whatsoever.

On examination, the right knee was still fully extendable, and there was slight crepitus on that side. The left knee was also slightly tender over the saphenous nerve. Both were again injected with the same gratifying results as before. She is still well and still playing tennis.

Mr. J. P. , aged 65, in the past had been a very keen sportsman, playing forward for Transvaal Rugby and participating in several international matches. He first came to my surgery walking with two sticks and assisted by two friends. During his previous sporting activities he had injured both knees many times and had undergone a menisectomy for his right knee in 1966, being told at the time he had arthritis. In 1981 he had a hernia operation, and after this the pain went to the left knee as well, which also became involved in osteoarthritis. After that he was never free of pain. Six months after his hernia operation he slipped on a Coca-Cola bottle, damaging his left knee very badly, and sustained a cracked fracture of his patella. This was treated conservatively by means of a plaster-of-paris cylinder. He also has mild hypertension and com- plains of dizziness, due possibly to an old neck injury which he received on the rugby field. He had previously been treated at the local hospital where he had been a regular attender due to concomitant hypertension for the past 15 years. He had also received treatment for his knee in the form of many anti- inflammatory drugs. Only one of these had any effect whatsoever, and this to no great extent. He had received treatment in the form of physiotherapy and was a regular attender at the local gymnasium in an effort to get himself more mobile.

He was only just able to get on the examination couch, and attempts at flexing the knee caused him considerable pain, There was also marked crepitus, which was worse in the left knee at the site of the old fractured patella, Flexion on either side was not possible for more than 25 degrees and stiffness was very marked. He was tender over the saphenous nerves, as well as over other neurological points asdescribed previously. These were injected by routine measures and at the conclusion of the procedure, both knees could be flexed easily to a right angle, and this was entirely painless. He was then asked to get off the couch and was able to do so and walked around the surgery unaided. He could not believe what had happened, and as he walked out into the waiting room his eyes were full of tears. He reattended two or three times for more injections, with further relief of his symptoms and increased mobility of his knees. After two weeks, he related that he was walking around as if in a dream, with no real pain. He had been able to go out dancing till well past midnight. He remains well to this day, only occasionally attending for further injections, and has become a very active member of the community.

CONCLUSION

In this short booklet, I have attempted to describe an easymethod for bringing under control the agony of arthritis of the knees. Not only does the method abolish pain but it is also harmless and possibly reverses the whole process.

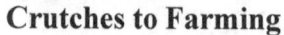

During the past six years, patients of all races have come to me from many corners of Southern Africa for relief of their pain. They attend once, twice or occasionally three times for their injections and then do not return for a year or more, their lives having been transformed. People formerly unable to play many forms of sport return to the golf course or bowling green or are able to go for medium-distance walks.Many are now able to plan overseas tripswhich before they could not contemplate. No longer is every step an agony; on the contrary, these previously partially disabled arthritics are now able to live a more than reasonable existence.

Crutches to Farming

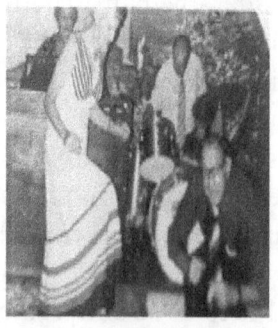

Many of my colleagues have been shown

this technique, and now use my method. Their results are also good. It is only a pity that even more do not do so, as they and their patients are missing so much.

Many experts will say that these results are purely subjective and anecdotal. This matters little in the long run, as what really concerns us all is that patients no longer have pain, and for this reason alone themethod is worth a trial. In the words of John Hunter:

Doing the Twist

References

1. Calandruccio RA. and Gilmer W. Scott. "Proflieration, regeneration and repair of articular cartilage of immature animals." *Surg.* 44-A (1962) 431-455.

2.Charcot J.M.,1875. "Lecons sur les Maladies du Systeme Nerveux." *Delahaye et cie.*, Paris. Vol. 1.

3.Crelin E.X. and Southwick W.D. "Changes induced by sustained pressure in the knee joint articular cartilage of adult rabbits." *Anat. Rac.* 149 (1964) 113-134.

4. Gowers W.R. and Taylor J., 1899. *Diseases of the Nervous System,* 3rd Edition, Churchill & Co., London.

5. Ignelzi R.J., Atkinson J.H., Pain and its Modulation 1. Afferent Mechanisms. *Neuro- Surgery*, 1980, 6, 577-583.

b. Iversen D I., lversen L.L. Substance P. "A new CNS transmitter." *Hospital Update*, 1981, 5, 497-506.

7. Lewis T., 1927. *Blood Vessels of the Human Skin*, Shaw and Co., London.

8. McCutchen C.E., "Animal joints and weeping lubrication." *New Scientist* 15 (1962) 412-415.

9. Mitchell S.W., Morehouse G.R., Keen W.W., 1864. *Gunshot Wounds and Other Injuries of Nerves*. Lippincott and Co., Philadelphia.

10. Salter R.S. and Field P. "The effects of continuous compression on living articular cartilage: An experimental investigation." *Journal Bone and Joint Surgery.* 42A (1960) 31-45.

11. Sollman T., 1957. *A Manual of Pharmacology,* 8th Edition. W.B. Saunders Co., Philadelphia.

12. Speransky A.D., 1935. *A basis for the theory of Medicine* International Publishers, N.Y.

13. Trias A. "Effect of persistent pressure on the articular cartilage: An experimental study." *Journal Bone and Joint Surgery.* 43B (1961) 476-386.

14. Wright S., 1952. *Applied Physiology,* 9th Edition, Oxford University Press, London. Page 721.

15. Wyburn-Mason R., 1978. *The Causation of Rheumatoid Disease and Many Human Cancers*. A New Concept in Medicine. Iji Publishing Co. Ltd., Tokyo, Japan.

16. _____,1964. *A New Protozoon*, Henry Kimpton, London.

17. _____, 1958. *The Reticulo-endothelial System in Growth and Tumour Formation,* Henry Kimpton, London.

18. _____,1949. *Trophic Nerves.* Henry Kimpton, London.

Injection Points for Intraneural Injections

Injection	Acupuncture	Nerve Root	Name of Nerve
#1	BL-9	C-2	Greater Occipital
#2	GB-11	C-2	Lesser Occipital
#3	BL-10	C-3	Third Occipital
#4	TH-23	Trigeminal	Zygomatic-Temporal
#5	BL-2	Trigeminal	Supraorbital
#6	SI-17	C-2,3	Great Auricular
#7	HT-1	C-5,6	Axillary (Lower Branch)
#8	Not Known	C-5,6	Axillary (Upper Branch) (Circum-flex humeral)
#9	TH-13	C-5,6	Lateral cutaneous of arm
#10	SI-9	C-5,6	Axillary bifurcation (Circumflex)
#11	SI-10	Brachial Plexus	Suprascapular
#12	C0-15	C-3,4	Suprascapular (Posterior Branch)
#13	TH-15	C-3,4	Suprascapular (Anterior Branch)
#14	BL-41	C-6,7,8	Thoracodorsal
#15	SI-12	C-5,6	Superior Subscapular
#16	LU-5	C-5,6,7	Lateral Cutaneous of forearm
#17	SI-8	C-8, T-1	Mediual Cutaneous of forearm
#18	HT-3	C-5,6,7,8, T-1	Median
#19	LU-8,9	C-5,6,7,8, T-1	Anterior Interosseous

#1 Lateral aspect of upper margin of external occipital protuber-
ance about 1 inch from midline

#2 On posterior aspect of mastoid process of temporal bone about
1-3/4" lateral to #1

#3 About 2" inferior to #1 and 3/4" lateral to midline

#4 Two centimeters above zygomatic arch at the lateral tip of the
eyebrow

#5 At the medial end of the eyebrow

#6 At point where juglar vein crosses anterior border of sternomas-
toid

#7 In mid axilla on medial aspect of axillary artery

#8 Just dorsal to anterior axillary fold or crease

#9 On posterior surface of arm approximately 1/2" lateral to
posterior axillary fold

#10 One thumbsbreath superior to posterior axillary fold

#11 Passing through suprascapular notch sending filaments to all
joints of shoulder

#12 Posterior-lateral and inferior to acrominion where depression
is formed with arm raised

#13 Superior over trapzius muscle 2 to 3 inches lateral to midline
at level of C-4

#14 Four fingerbreadths (of patients) or 3-1/2" lateral to inferior
end of spinous process T2

#15 In middle of superspinatus fossa

#16 At cubital fossa on the radial aspect of triceps tendon

#17 Anterior to medial epicondyle of humerous with elbow flexed
(Maybe found as the nerve merges through the deep fascia
in front of media epicondyle)

#18 F-3 Never used

#19 Never used

Injection Points for Intraneural Injections (Continued)

Injection	Acupuncture	Nerve Root	Name of Nerve
#20	TH-24	C-5,6,7,8, T-1	Posterior Interosseous Ganglion
#21	CO-4	C-5,6,7,8, T-1	Radial Terminal Branches
#22	SP-20	T-2,3	Lateral Pectoral Nerves
	SP-21	T-5	Lateral Cutaneous
#23	KS-27	T-1	Anterior Cutaneous
	KJ-26	T-2	Anterior Cutaneous
	KJ-25	T-3	Anterior Cutaneous
	KJ-24	T-4	Anterior Cutaneous
	KJ-23	T-4	Anterior Cutaneous
	KJ-22	T-4	Anterior Cutaneous
#24	BL-27	S-1	Posterior Rami S-1
	BL-28	S-2	Posterior Rami S-2
	BL-29	S-3	Posterior Rami S-3
#25	BL-30	S-4	Posterior Rami S-4
#26	BL-35	S-5	Postrior Rami S-5
#27	BL-37	S-1,2,3	Posterior Femoral
#28	GB-27,28	L-2,3	Lateral Femoral Cutaneous
#29	L1-11	L-2,3,4	Acessory Obturator
#30A	None Known	L-2,3,4	Obturator
#30B			Nerve to Rectus Femoris
#39C			Nerve to Qudratus Femoris
#31	GB-30		Joint Capsule (Hip)
#32	ST-34	L-2,3,4	Intemediate Femoral Cutaneous

#20 On the dorsum of the wrist in the depression of the skin crease proximal to the third and fourth metacarpals

#21 On dorsum of hand in anatomical snuff box

#22 Six inches lateral to mid sternal line at a line even with the intercostal space

#22 In the mid axillary line in the sixth intercoastal space

#23 One and 3/4 inches lateral to mid sternal line in the 1st intercoastal space

One and 3/4 inches lateral to mid sternal line in the 2nd intercoastal space

One and 3/4 inches lateral to mid sternal line in the 3rd intercoastal space

One and 3/4 inches lateral to mid sternal line in the 4th intercoastal space

One and 3/4 inches lateral to mid sternal line in the 5th intercoastal space

One and 3/4 inches lateral to mid sternal line in the 6th intercoastal space . . . Etc.

#24 One to one and one half inches lateral to 1st sacral vertebrae joint

One to two inches lateral to 2nd sacral vertebrae, superior to sacral iliac joint

One to two inches lateral to 3rd sacral vertebrae level with anterior superior crest of the ilium

#25 One to two inches lateral to sacral hiatus

#26 One centimeter lateral to the midline of spine level with the superior border of the coccyx

#27 Trigger points can be anywhere in a two inch brand running down the mid posterior thigh from the gluteal region to the back of the knee

#28 Anterior and about one inch inferior to the anteior superior spine of the ilium

#29 Approximaterly one inch inferior to medial end of Poupart's ligament

#30A Anterior area of greater trochanter. Insert needle at X and penetrate to trochanter

#30B Superior area of greater trochanter. Insert needle at X and penetrate to trochanter

#30C Posterior area of greater trochanter. Insert needle at X and penetrate to trochanter

#31 Two thirds of distance from midline on a line joining the greater trochanter with sacral hiatus

#32 Two to three thumbsbreadths superior to the patella along the lateral margin of the patella

Injection Points for Intraneural Injections (Continued)

Injection	Acupuncture	Nerve Root	Name of Nerve
#33	SP-10	L-2,3,4	Medial Femoral Cutaneous
#34	SP-11	L-2,3,4	Saphenous #1 femoral canal
#35	OB-31,32	L-2,3	Lateral Femoral Cutaneous
#36	SP-9	L-2,3,4	Saphenous
#37	?	L-2,3,4	Saphenous
#38	?	L-2,3 ,4	Saphenous
#39	?	L-2,3,4	Saphenous
#40	ST-36	L-4,5	Musculocutaneous (Peroneal)
#41	SP-6	L-2,3,4	Saphenous for Foot
#42	L1-4	L-2,3,4	Saphenous for Foot
#43	ST-41	L-4,5 S-1,2	Anterior Tibial (Deep Perineal)
#44	Bl-59,60	L-4,5 S-1,2,3	Sural

Location of Tender and Injection Points nd Details of Possible Variations

#33 Two thusbreadths superior to the medial border of the patella on the
medial aspect of the thigh

#34 Approximately 6 inches superior to #33 in medial aspect of Sartorius

#35 On the lateral aspect of the thigh approximately four to six inches
proximal to the superior border of the patella

#36 At attachment of median longitudinal ligament 1-2 centimeters to
'medial condyle of tibia about 1 inch medial to patella. This point
often relieves ankle pain.

#37 At origin of infrapatellar branch of the nerve

#38 Immediately below the patella. There may be two to three points
located here.

#39 At the apex of the curve in the nerve as it enters the subcutaneous
tissues

#40 Approximately 3 inches inferior to tibial tuberosity an done finger
lateral to crest of finger in the tibialis muscle

#41 At the junction of mid and lower 1/3 of the shaft of tibia approximately
4 inches superior to apex to the medial malleolus ana slightly
medial to tibial crest

#42 At the lower 1/4 of the tibial shaft two thumbs superior to the medial
malleolus and lying just medial to the tibial crest

#43 On dorsum of the foot in the center of the inferior extensor retenaculum and
between the tendons of the extensor hellicus longus and extensor
digitorium longus

#44 In the depression antior to the Achilles Tendon and posterior to the
lateral malleolus
Also three inches superior to this point

Nerve Sites for Intraneural Injection

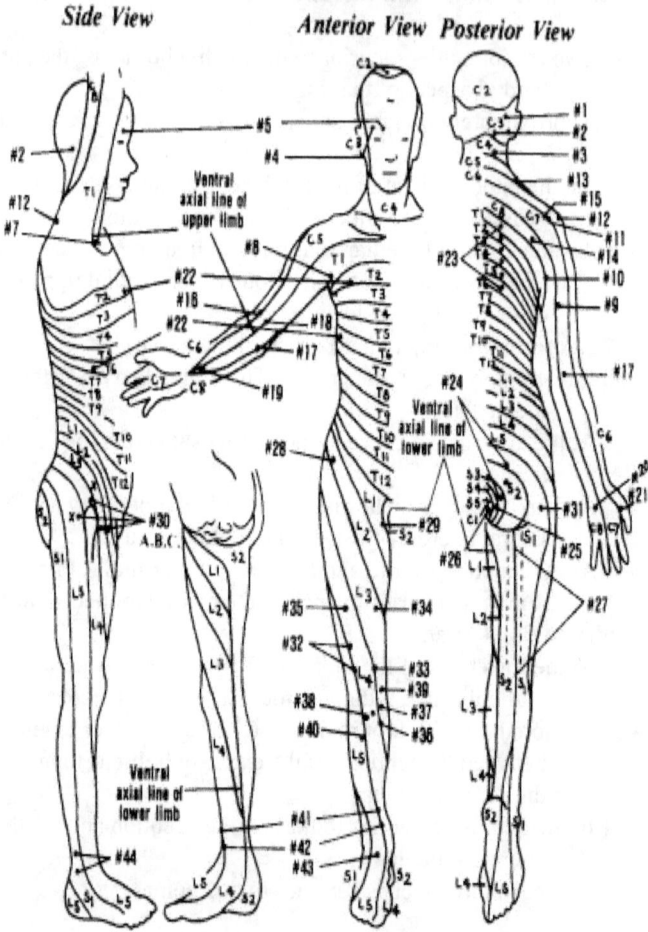

Side View **Anterior View** **Posterior View**

Schematic Drawing II

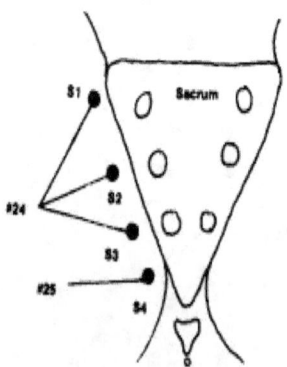

Points for Sciatica